14.99

MORECAMBE BAY HOSPITALS NHS TRUST

**Comments on *Type 1 Diabetes: Answers at your fingertips*
from readers:**

'It's a great book! I've learned a lot from it. I have read previous
editions, and much prefer this Sixth Edition, which has a book
especially for Type 1s like me – and tells me things I need to know.'

J H,
Bristol

D1078201

Comments on earlier editions from readers

'An excellent book. It is comprehensive, informative, and easy to read and understand.'

DON KENDRICK,
Seaton, Devon

'A marvellous book – just what the layman needs.'

MRS P PILLEY,
Hornchurch

'I like the form it takes (questions and answers); it makes it much easier to find the specific areas when a problem does arise. Also it makes easier reading for picking up and putting down without having to wade through chapter after chapter of heavy medical jargon which for the lay person can be very difficult to take in and understand.'

MRS PAM MUNFORD,
Lincoln

'I have read the book myself from cover to cover and found it to be most informative, up-to-date and presented in a format which is easy to assimilate by the majority of people with diabetes who will undoubtedly relate some question to a particular experience of their own – and find the answer.'

PHILIP WHITMORE,
Macclesfield

'I think the book is excellent value since it answers all the basic questions of diabetes and has answers to questions I have not seen written down before. (In fact the whole family is interested in reading it.)'

D BALL,
Nottingham

Reviews of previous editions

'Overall this is a most interesting and useful book suitable for people with diabetes, their families, health professionals and anyone interested in diabetes. It is a book that once bought will be used over and over again, and works out to be good value.'

BALANCE

'. . . a guide, in lively question and answer form, to coping with diabetes. It is quite possible to lead a full life providing the sufferer understands and can control the disease.'

WOMAN'S JOURNAL

'Has positive information to help both young and old lead active lives with the minimum of restrictions.'

GOOD HOUSEKEEPING

'I would recommend it to people living with diabetes, but also to professionals in the diabetes field.'

PROFESSIONAL NURSE

'The book is well presented, with good, clear illustrations and is reasonably priced. I highly recommend it for people newly diagnosed with diabetes and their families and as a source of reference for nurses dealing with diabetes.'

NURSING STANDARD

'Woe betide any clinicians or nurses whose patients have read this invaluable source of down-to-earth information when they have not.'

THE LANCET

*This sixth edition is dedicated to Peter Sönksen
and Sue Judd whose inspiration and energy
led to the first edition of the book.*

Type 1 Diabetes

Answers at your fingertips

SIXTH EDITION

Charles Fox BM, FRCP

*Consultant Physician with
Special Interest in Diabetes,
Northampton General Hospital*

Anne Kilvert MD, FRCP

*Consultant Physician with
Special Interest in Diabetes,
Northampton General Hospital*

MORECAMBE BAY HOSPITALS NHS TRUST

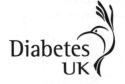

Diabetes
UK

The charity for
people with diabetes
is pleased to have worked
with Class Publishing
on this book

CLASS PUBLISHING · LONDON

© Peter Sönksen, Charles Fox, Sue Judd 1991, 1992, 1994, 1997, 1998, 1999, 2001, 2002, 2003

© Charles Fox, Anne Kilvert, 2008

All rights reserved

The authors assert their right as set out in Sections 77 and 78 of the Copyright Designs and Patents Act 1988 to be identified as the authors of this work wherever it is published commercially and whenever any adaptation of this work is published or produced including any sound recordings or films made of or based upon this work.

Printing history
First published as *Diabetes at Your Fingertips* 1985, reprinted 1987
Second edition, 1991
Reprinted with revisions 1991 and 1992
Third edition,1994
Reprinted 1995, 1996, with revisions 1997
Fourth edition, 1998
Reprinted with revisions 1999, 2002, 2003
Sixth edition (as two books, *Type 1 Diabetes* and *Type 2 Diabetes*) 2008

The authors and publishers welcome feedback from the users of this book. Please contact the publishers.

Class Publishing, Barb House, Barb Mews, London W6 7PA, UK
Telephone: 020 7371 2119
Fax: 020 7371 2878 [International +4420] 616. 462
email: post@class.co.uk Fox
Website: www.class.co.uk

A CIP catalogue for this book is available from the British Library

ISBN 978 1 85959 175 8

10 9 8 7 6 5 4 3 2 1

Edited by Caroline Sheldrick

Cartoons by Jane Taylor

Line illustrations by David Woodroffe

Designed and typeset by Martin Bristow

Printed and bound In Finland by WS Bookwell, Juva

Contents

Foreword

by **Sir Steve Redgrave** CBE
Vice-President, Diabetes UK

Diabetes: Answers at your fingertips has always – in its five editions, published over 20 years – shown a very constructive and positive approach to dealing with diabetes. Its layout encourages readers to develop a good understanding of their condition and to question their approach to the disease.

This new Sixth Edition maintains the same positive approach, and is now in two parallel versions: one specifically for people with Type 1 diabetes, the other written for people with Type 2 diabetes.

I have no hesitation in commending this book, which helps towards our understanding of diabetes as well as being very constructive in dealing with issues that surround the condition. I have always maintained that 'I have diabetes but it doesn't have me.' As well as going out and leading a very active and normal life, not allowing diabetes to restrain you in any way, learning more about diabetes is also very positive. Happy reading.

Foreword

Peter Sönksen and Sue Judd
Co-authors of previous editions

After 20 years with *Diabetes at your fingertips*, we were delighted to read this new book and to be invited to write a Foreword. Sensibly, the authors and publishers have decided that it would now be better to have two versions designed specifically for Type 1 and 2 diabetes.

This book will be of great value to people with Type 1 diabetes, as well as to any of their friends and family who wish to explore the condition and its treatment in more detail. It will also be invaluable to the professional medical and paramedical staff responsible for delivering care to people with diabetes, particularly those in the community.

Written in the now familiar 'questions and answers' format, it is designed for dipping into rather than cover-to-cover reading, but newly diagnosed patients might well like to read its contents *in toto* and will benefit from doing so.

The secret to successful self-care is knowledge, confidence and motivation; this new book will make a significant, positive contribution to this important area.

Peter Sönksen MD, FRCP, FFSEM (UK)
Emeritus Professor of Endocrinology

Sue Judd SRN
Retired Diabetes Specialist Nurse
St Thomas' Hospital, London

Preface

Is this the right book for you? Do you have Type 1 diabetes?

This is the sixth edition of *Diabetes: Answers at your fingertips* and in this new edition, we have made some important changes. The original book was designed to answer questions about both Type 1 and Type 2 diabetes. In the new version, we have decided to write separate books for each type of diabetes and this book is for people with Type 1.

You may not be sure which type of diabetes you have. There is a general rule that people with Type 1 diabetes are usually young, tend to be underweight at the time of diagnosis and need treatment with insulin straight away. However, the rule does not always apply: people can develop Type 1 diabetes at any age and are not always underweight.

If your diabetes needed insulin treatment from the time of diagnosis or if you failed to respond to tablets, this book is for you.

Acknowledgements

We are grateful to all the people who helped in the production of past editions of *Diabetes at your fingertips*: Anna Fox, Peter Swift, Clara Lowy, Suzanne Lucas and Judith North.

Peter Sönksen and Sue Judd had the original idea of a question and answer book for people with diabetes (*The Diabetes Reference Book*). This new edition is based on their text and the clear practical advice they gave.

We thank the following writers for their contributions to the new edition: Florence Brown for providing the nursing perspective in the chapters on insulin and monitoring; Helen Millar for answers to the questions on diet; Chris Moudiotis for advice about diabetes in children; Maria Mousley for the podiatry section and Liz Robinson for advice on the questions on alcohol.

We would like to thank the people who reviewed the book and provided helpful advice: Peter Sönksen and Sue Judd, Vasso Vydelingum for a cultural perspective, Peter Lapsley, Julia Harkess, Claire Mehmet and finally Rosie Walker for a detailed critique.

Our editors Caroline Sheldrick and Richenda Milton-Thompson have been both encouraging and endlessly patient. Jane Taylor drew the new cartoons. Richard Warner of Class Publishing has been the driving force.

Introduction

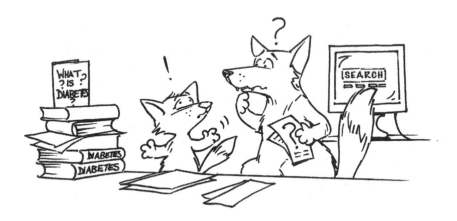

You may be reading this because you, or someone close to you, have been found to have Type 1 diabetes. If you have just discovered that you have diabetes, you will probably feel shocked and anxious. There will be no time to adjust to the news before you have to make major alterations in lifestyle, with the need for insulin injections, blood tests and changes in what you eat. A lot of people, nurses, dietitians, doctors and podiatrists, will give you information and it may difficult to take it all in. Diabetes is a complicated condition and it will take time to learn everything you need to know – don't feel pressured to learn it all at once.

Living with diabetes involves making day-to-day decisions which can only be made by you (or by parents of a child with diabetes). A lot of effort is being put into diabetes education so that people can make well-informed decisions. We hope this book will add to the education you receive and allow you to look up the answers as questions occur to you.

Remember that no one involved in diabetes, including healthcare professionals, ever stops learning more about it.

How to use this book

Most chapters comprise a series of questions and answers, and are not designed to be read from beginning to end. However, some chapters could well be read through at the outset, in particular Chapter 1: **What is diabetes?**, Chapter 4: **Monitoring and control**, and Chapter 9: **Long-term complications**.

If you are newly diagnosed, you may not be ready to come to grips with Chapter 10: **Research and the future** but you may want to discover what is known about the causes of diabetes (in Chapter 1). If you have just started insulin injections you should read the following sections at an early stage.

- Hypos (in Chapter 3)

- Other illnesses (in Chapter 5)

- Types of insulin (in Chapter 3)

- Blood glucose monitoring (in Chapter 4)

- Driving (in Chapter 5)

- Emergencies (Chapter 12)

People who have lived with diabetes for several years will want to check whether our answers in Chapter 5: **Life with diabetes** agree with their own experience.

Feedback is the most important feature of good diabetes care. This relies on people being honest with doctors, nurses and dietitians and vice versa. Not everyone will agree with every answer we give, but the book can only be improved if you let us know if you have found our advice to be unhelpful. We would also like to know if there are important questions that we have not covered. Please write to us c/o Class Publishing, Barb House, Barb Mews, London W6 7PA, UK or email: post@class.co.uk.

1 | What is diabetes?

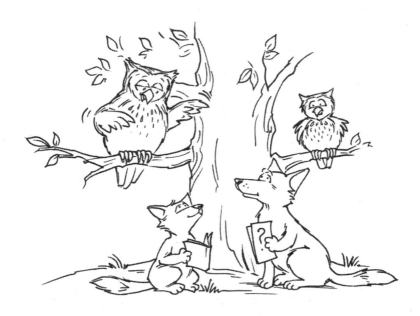

In this chapter we describe the central problem in diabetes, which is an increase in the amount of glucose (sugar) in the blood. We explain why this happens and why it may be dangerous.

There are two main types of diabetes.

- Type 1 – this type of diabetes usually appears in younger people under the age of 40 but may occur at any age. It is treated by insulin injections and diet.

- Type 2 – this type of diabetes usually appears in people over the age of 40. They may have had undetected diabetes for many years and may not feel particularly unwell. Diabetes in older people is often discovered by chance and commonly responds well to diet or tablets, although with the passage of time, most people need insulin therapy.

There are other rare types of diabetes, which we also mention in this chapter.

WHAT HAPPENS IN DIABETES?

The pancreas is a gland situated in the upper part of the abdomen and connected by a fine tube to the intestine (see Figure 1.1). One of its functions is to release into the gut digestive juices, which are mixed with food soon after it leaves the stomach.

These digestive juices are needed to break down food and help it be absorbed into the body. This part of the pancreas has nothing to do with diabetes.

The pancreas also produces a number of hormones which are released directly into the bloodstream, unlike the digestive juices which pass into the intestine. The most important of these hormones is insulin, a shortage of which causes diabetes. The other important

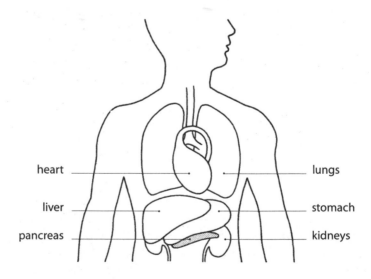

Figure 1.1 Location of the pancreas

hormone produced by the pancreas is glucagon, which has the opposite action to insulin and may be used in correcting serious hypos. 'Hypo' is short for hypoglycaemia, meaning low blood glucose. See the section *Hypos* in Chapter 3. Both hormones come from a part of the pancreas called the islets of Langerhans, which are scattered throughout the pancreas.

Why does the body need insulin?

Without insulin the body cannot make use of the food we eat. Food is broken down in the stomach and intestine into simple chemicals, such as glucose and fatty acids, which provide fuel for all the activities of the body. These simple chemicals also provide building blocks for growth or replacing worn out parts, and any extra is stored for later use. In diabetes, food is broken down as normal but, because of the shortage of insulin (or sometimes because insulin does not work properly), excess glucose cannot be stored and builds up in the bloodstream. When glucose rises above a certain level, it spills into the urine through the kidneys.

The liver plays a dual role in processing food. It converts simple chemicals into complex substances which are then stored for future use and it also allows breakdown of these stores when they are needed for fuel. This process is controlled by insulin. For example, in the absence of insulin, glycogen (starch) is broken down into glucose, which pours out of the liver into the bloodstream (and then into the urine). Insulin switches off this outpouring of glucose and causes the glucose to be stored as glycogen. Thus insulin ensures that a perfect balance is kept between the production of glucose and its storage, and in this way it maintains the blood glucose at a normal level. Insulin plays other important roles, such as allowing glucose to get into other parts of the body to be used as a fuel, and regulating the processing of amino acids and fatty acids, which are the breakdown products of protein and fat.

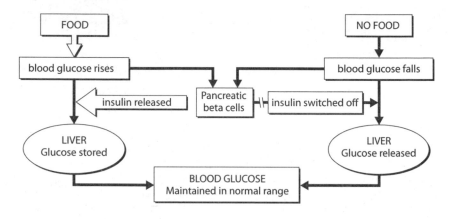

Figure 1.2 Insulin production system

What happens to insulin production in diabetes?

In people who do not have diabetes, insulin is produced in the pancreas and released into the blood as soon as the blood glucose level starts to rise after eating. Insulin travels straight from the pancreas to the liver where it has the important role of regulating glucose production and the storage of glucose as glycogen. The level of glucose in the blood then falls and, as it does so, insulin production is switched off, allowing glucose to be released from stores in the liver (see Figure 1.2). In people who do not have diabetes this sensitive system keeps the amount of glucose in the blood at a steady level.

In diabetes this process is faulty. People with Type 2 diabetes can still produce some insulin but not in adequate amounts to keep the blood glucose level normal. This is because their insulin does not work properly (a condition called 'insulin resistance'). People with Type 1 diabetes have little or no insulin of their own and need injections of insulin to try to keep the blood glucose level normal. Even if given four or five times a day, injected insulin is not as efficient at regulating blood glucose as the pancreas, which responds instantly to small changes in blood glucose by switching the insulin supply on or off.

There are three main factors affecting the level of glucose in the blood:

- food (which puts it up);

- insulin (which brings it down);

- exercise (which also brings it down).

Any form of stress, such as an illness like flu, increases blood glucose. Learning how to balance your blood glucose level in diabetes is a matter of trial and error. This involves taking a lot of blood glucose measurements and discovering how various foods and forms of exercise affect the levels.

TYPES OF DIABETES

I hadn't realised that there were different types of diabetes until I was diagnosed recently. What are the different types?

Diabetes does exist in different forms. Two main types are recognised.

- Type 1 diabetes usually occurs in younger people. This condition develops suddenly and insulin injections are nearly always needed as soon as it is diagnosed. About one in ten of all people with diabetes fall into this category, which used to be called 'insulin dependent diabetes'.

- Type 2 diabetes usually occurs in older people, who are often overweight, and have less obvious symptoms. Obesity is linked to insulin resistance, which is a root cause of Type 2 diabetes and insulin resistance occurs many years before diabetes itself begins. As the population becomes more overweight, Type 2 diabetes is developing in younger age groups, including children. At the onset of Type 2 diabetes, treatment is with diet with or without tablets. After a few years, people with Type 2 diabetes nearly always need to use insulin, because of the progressive nature of this condition.

I have been told that I have diabetes insipidus. Is this the same as the diabetes that my friend's elderly father has?

The only connection between diabetes insipidus and the more common form of diabetes (where the full name is diabetes mellitus) is that people with both conditions pass large amounts of urine. Diabetes insipidus is a rare condition caused by an abnormality in the pituitary gland and not the pancreas. One disorder does not lead to the other, and diabetes insipidus does not carry the risk of long-term complications found in diabetes mellitus.

CAUSES OF DIABETES

Despite a vast amount of research throughout the world the cause of diabetes is not known. Some families carry an extra risk of diabetes (see the section *Inheritance* on p. 9).

I have developed Type 1 diabetes. Is there anything I could have done to prevent this happening to me?

If you are the only member of your close family with diabetes, there is nothing you could have done to prevent it. If you have a parent or sibling (brother or sister) with Type 1 diabetes, it is possible that your risk of diabetes could have been predicted. Even so, we do not know of any way of preventing Type 1 diabetes from developing in those people at risk.

A number of research groups have looked at ways of preventing diabetes in people at risk. One such study, based in Oxford, looked at the siblings and parents of children with Type 1 diabetes. Some of the siblings had antibodies to the cells in the pancreas which produce insulin (islet cell antibodies) and these children had a much higher risk of developing diabetes. The children at risk were treated with the drug nicotinamide as it was thought that this might reduce the risk of diabetes. Unfortunately the results were disappointing: nicotinamide did not protect children from diabetes. So at present, although it may be possible to identify young people who are at risk of developing Type 1 diabetes, there is no way of preventing this from happening, once damage to the insulin cells is in progress.

Could diabetes be triggered by a virus?

Some scientists used to suspect that a certain virus could be the cause of diabetes in young people but proof is lacking and this theory now seems very unlikely to be true.

There is certainly no 'diabetes virus' and you cannot catch diabetes in the same way as chickenpox.

Is diabetes a disease of modern times?

The earliest detailed description of diabetes was made more than 2000 years ago but it is much more common now than in the past. This is particularly true of Type 2 diabetes, which is becoming very common in some countries such as India. Diabetes in younger people is also becoming more common, and this has been related to increasing affluence and obesity. Type 1 diabetes is also becoming more common, particularly in children under five years old. The reasons are not well understood.

My mother died very suddenly last year and not long afterwards I was diagnosed with diabetes. Can a bad shock bring on diabetes?

Sometimes diabetes develops soon after a major disturbance in life, such as a bereavement, a heart attack or a bad accident, and the diabetes is blamed on the upset. This is not really the case, as insulin failure in the pancreas takes a long time to develop. However, a bad shock can stress the system and bring on diabetes a bit earlier if your insulin supply is already running low.

> *I developed diabetes in my last pregnancy and was told it would go away once the baby was born. This did not happen and I still need to take insulin injections. Why is this?*

Most women who develop diabetes in pregnancy are at risk of developing Type 2 diabetes later in life. Occasionally, women who are in the process of developing Type 1 diabetes become pregnant and the diabetes comes to light sooner. This is because pregnancy places greater demands on the pancreas and the effects of insulin deficiency become obvious at an earlier stage. Diabetes and pregnancy are dealt with in detail in Chapter 7.

> *I have had to go to hospital for repeated attacks of pancreatitis and now have diabetes. I am told that these two conditions are related – is this true?*

Pancreatitis can be a very painful and unpleasant illness: it means that your pancreas has become inflamed. The pancreas is the gland that produces insulin as well as other hormones and digestive juices. If it is severely inflamed or damaged, it may not be able to produce enough insulin. Sometimes diabetes develops during or after an attack of pancreatitis and tablets or insulin are needed to keep control of the blood glucose. This form of diabetes is usually, but not always, permanent.

> *What other diseases would increase the chances of getting Type 1 diabetes?*

Type 1 diabetes is one of a group of conditions known as autoimmune disorders because the body attacks various organs and interferes with their normal function. Proteins called antibodies are formed against specific parts of the body, including endocrine glands

(glands which produce hormones). The antibodies interfere with hormone production and usually lead to a failure of that particular gland. In Type 1 diabetes antibodies are formed against the islet cells of the pancreas, which are responsible for producing insulin. Other examples of autoimmune endocrine disorders are thyroid disease (both underactive and overactive) and Addison's Disease (adrenal gland failure). Other autoimmune conditions associated with Type 1 diabetes include pernicious anaemia (failure to absorb vitamin B12), coeliac disease (gluten sensitivity) and vitiligo (a disorder of skin pigmentation). Although this group of conditions are linked by a similar underlying cause, it is very uncommon for any one person to have more than two of these disorders. However, they often run in families.

Inheritance

My father had Type 1 diabetes. Am I likely to get it too?

Type 1 diabetes occurs in about three people per 1000 – it is ten times less common than Type 2 diabetes. It is sometimes possible to identify people at increased risk of Type 1 diabetes, using genetic tests. However, these are not easy to carry out and in practice are only used in research projects. Surprisingly it is not easy to find figures for the exact risk you have of inheriting diabetes from your father. Most experts agree that the risk is between 5 and 10%. For some unexplained reason, the risk would be much lower if your mother had diabetes – only 2–3%. If both your parents had diabetes, your risk of having Type 1 diabetes might be as high as 30%. Despite this family risk, Type 1 diabetes does not usually run in families and only about 10% of people with Type 1 diabetes have a close relative with this condition.

In some cases, we have known parents who develop Type 1 diabetes some years after their child as if the genetics was working backwards! The child then becomes the role model for the parent.

I come from an Indian family and number of my relatives have diabetes. I have been told that diabetes is more common in Asian families. Is this true?

It is an unfortunate fact that diabetes is much more common in families who originate from the Indian subcontinent, but this is usually Type 2 diabetes. The risk seems to be related to moving from a subsistence life, where people have to work hard in order to grow enough food for survival, to a comparatively easy life of relative affluence, where food is easily available and hard physical work is no longer a fact of life. Indians who live in an urban environment have a risk of diabetes up to five times greater than that of a white person with a similar lifestyle. People of Indian origin who live in this country must be aware of their risk of diabetes, especially if parents and relatives are affected. As in all cases of diabetes, early diagnosis is vital if complications are going to be avoided.

I've been told that people from certain parts of the world are more at risk of diabetes. Could you tell me more about this?

It is well known that certain populations, such as South Asians, are at increased risk of Type 2 diabetes. The risk of Type 1 diabetes is less related to racial origin but varies with latitude. Thus the closer you go to the North Pole, the greater the risk of diabetes. So there are more children with diabetes in Scotland and Sweden than those who live near the Mediterranean. The curious exception is Sardinia, which has one of the highest rates of Type 1 diabetes in the world.

Several members of my family developed diabetes when we were young and most of us are controlled by tablets. I've been told we are a MODY family. What does this mean?

MODY stands for Maturity-Onset Diabetes of the Young. (Maturity-onset diabetes is an earlier name for Type 2 diabetes.) In the 1970s, it was noticed that a handful of families seemed to develop diabetes in their teens or twenties and about 50% of family members were affected. This suggests a certain sort of inheritance (autosomal dominant); those family members with diabetes have a specific defect in their insulin-producing cells. Research into these people with diabetes has increased our understanding of the causes of diabetes. There are several distinct types of MODY, but generally people in this group can control their diabetes with tablets and do not usually need insulin. However, because this type of diabetes occurs in young people, it may be mistaken for Type 1 diabetes and wrongly treated with insulin. Visit the website: www.projects.ex.ac.uk/diabetesgenes/mody/index.htm to find out more about this unusual form of diabetes.

If diabetes is known to be in my family, should I or my children take any preventive action?

The inheritance of diabetes is a complicated subject and different types of diabetes are inherited in different ways. In Type 1 diabetes some family members may carry an increased risk, which can be identified by genetic testing. However, only a small proportion of the people who inherit this risk will go on to develop diabetes and no one has been able to pin down the factors that cause this to happen. A number of research projects have tried different treatments to prevent diabetes in family members identified as being at risk, but sadly these have all been unsuccessful. As there is no known way of preventing diabetes in such people and because the individual risk is small, genetic testing is only done as part of a research project.

Type 2 diabetes is more strongly inherited than Type 1, and therefore often affects several members of the same family. It is now clear that a number of different genes are involved. The picture which is slowly emerging suggests that there are several different forms of Type 2 diabetes. The genetics of one rare form of inherited diabetes, called MODY, have been investigated in great detail and have increased our understanding of this condition but these discoveries do not apply to the vast majority of people with Type 2 diabetes (see MODY question above).

There is now evidence that family members who are at risk may put off developing diabetes by regular exercise, losing weight and sometimes by taking medication. They should have a blood glucose test as soon as they develop any relevant symptoms, so that diabetes can be detected and treated early.

I am 16 and have had diabetes for five years. Why has my identical twin brother not got diabetes?

A large 20-year research project has studied examples of identical twins with diabetes. The results show a difference between the way Type 1 and Type 2 diabetes are inherited. If you have an identical twin with Type 1 diabetes, you have only a 50% chance of developing diabetes yourself. On the other hand, if you had Type 2 diabetes (extremely unusual at the age of 11) your twin would be almost certain to get the same sort of diabetes. If your twin brother has not developed diabetes within the last five years, he has a very low risk of developing the condition.

SYMPTOMS

My 11-year-old son suddenly became very thirsty and was diagnosed with diabetes. What is the cause of the thirst?

The first signs of diabetes in a young person are thirst and loss of weight. These two symptoms are related and one leads to the other (there is more detail on weight loss in the answer to the next question). The first thing to go wrong is the increased amount of urine. Normally we pass about 1.5 litres (about 2 pints) of urine per day but people with uncontrolled diabetes may produce five times that amount. The continual loss of fluid dries out the body and the sensation of thirst is a warning that, unless they drink enough to replace the extra urine, they will soon become very dehydrated.

Of course people who do not have diabetes may also pass large amounts of urine. Most beer drinkers know the effects of five pints of bitter. In this case it is the volume of beer that causes the extra urine, whereas in diabetes the large volume of urine causes the thirst. In the early stages, the thirst is usually mild and most people fail to realise its significance unless they have had some personal experience of diabetes. Someone with undiagnosed diabetes will often take jugs of water up to bed, wake in the night to quench their thirst and pass urine, and still not realise that something is wrong. It would be helpful if more people knew that troublesome thirst may be due to diabetes.

I had lost quite a lot of weight before I was finally diagnosed with diabetes. Why was this?

The main fuel for the body is glucose, which is obtained from the digestion of sugary or starchy food. People with untreated diabetes cannot use this glucose as fuel or store it in the normal way. The unused glucose builds up in their bloodstream and overflows into the urine. Someone who has uncontrolled diabetes may lose as much as 500 g (just over 1 lb) of glucose (sugar) in their urine in 24 hours. Anyone trying to lose weight knows that sugar equals calories. These calories contained in the urine are lost to the body and are a drain on its resources. The 500 g of glucose lost are equivalent to 10 currant buns (2 000 calories per day).

Lack of insulin means that the body cannot use glucose to provide energy or to build stores of starch and fat. As a result body tissues are broken down to form glucose and ketones (see the section *Urine* in Chapter 4), and this causes loss of fat and wasting of muscles.

My vagina has been really itchy and sore. My GP says it's to do with my diabetes. Can this be right?

A woman whose diabetes is out of control may be troubled by itching around the vagina. The technical name for this distressing symptom is pruritus vulvae. The equivalent complaint may be seen in men when the end of the penis becomes sore (balanitis). If the foreskin is also affected, it may become thickened (phimosis), which prevents the foreskin from being pulled back and makes it difficult to keep the penis clean.

These problems are the result of infection (commonly known as thrush) from certain yeasts, especially *Candida*, which thrive on the high concentration of glucose in this region. If you keep your urine free from glucose by good control of your diabetes, the itching and soreness will normally clear up. Anti-yeast cream from your doctor or pharmacist may speed up the improvement but this is only a holding measure while glucose is cleared from your urine.

I have had blurred vision for a few weeks and have just been found to have diabetes. Why has this affected my vision?

The lens of the eye is responsible for focusing the image on the retina. Blurred vision is usually a temporary change, which can be corrected by wearing glasses. The lens of the eye becomes swollen when diabetes is out of control and this leads to long-sightedness. As the diabetes comes under control the lens of the eye returns to normal. A pair of glasses fitted for a swollen lens at a time of uncontrolled diabetes will no longer be suitable when the diabetes is brought under control. If you have been newly diagnosed with diabetes and find that you have blurred vision, you should wait for a few weeks after the glucose levels have fallen before visiting an optician for new spectacles. The blurred vision may improve on its own and new glasses may not be needed.

Most of the serious eye problems caused by diabetes are due to damage to the retina (retinopathy). The retina is the 'photographic plate' at the back of the eye. Even minor changes in the retina take several years to develop but older people may have diabetes for years without being aware of it. In such cases the retina may already be damaged by the time diabetes is diagnosed.

In very rare cases the lens of the eye may be permanently damaged (cataract) when diabetes is badly out of control. This can be treated by removing the cataract and replacing it with an artificial lens.

See the section *Eyes* in Chapter 9.

Can diabetes be discovered by chance?

Yes, but this usually happens only in Type 2 diabetes. In Type 1 diabetes the diagnosis is more likely to be made because someone feels unwell and goes to the doctor.

In older people with no obvious medical problems, diabetes is often discovered as a result of a routine urine test – for example in the course of an insurance examination. Once the diagnosis is made, the person may realise that they have been feeling slightly thirsty or tired, but these symptoms may be so mild that they go unnoticed. However, even people who have had very few symptoms often feel they have more energy once diabetes is controlled.

Sometimes people are found to have diabetes when they suffer another medical condition such as a heart attack or a foot infection. In such cases diabetes, previously undiagnosed, has been the main cause of the new problem. The important message is that even though the symptoms may be minor, so-called 'mild' diabetes may lead to serious problems.

2 | Diet and lifestyle

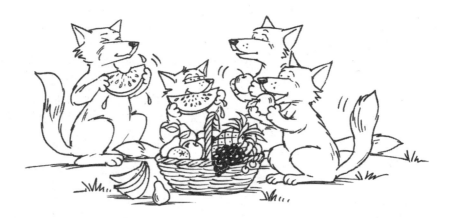

Type 1 diabetes is treated with a combination of diet and insulin. In this chapter we describe the dietary and lifestyle advice you need to control your diabetes. The next chapter will address the question of how to use insulin to keep the blood glucose normal.

Most people with diabetes, and especially parents who have a child with diabetes, long for a miracle cure. This explains why we have been sent so many questions about unorthodox methods of treatment. We have tried to answer these questions in a sensitive manner but there is no escaping the fact that, for a child, insulin is the only 'miracle cure' and that is how it was regarded when it was discovered in 1921.

Whether you have Type 1 or Type 2 diabetes, the most important thing is to access good diabetes education. In the past, people were often given instructions about what to eat without any explanation as to why it was important. Not surprisingly, they did not always follow the advice. The importance of structured education has been recognised in the Diabetes National Service Framework (NSF, see p. 124) and education programmes have been developed for both Type 1 and Type 2 diabetes. An example of structured education for Type 1 diabetes is the DAFNE programme (Dose Adjustment For Normal Eating) and you can read about this in the section *Why monitor?* in Chapter 4.

DIABETES EDUCATION

My doctor has just told me that I have Type 1 diabetes and I have started insulin with the help of the specialist nurse. I am very shocked and confused and feel that my life has been turned upside down. There seems to be such a lot to learn and I wonder how I am going to cope. My doctor has given me the phone number of Diabetes UK so I can get more information but I would really like to talk to someone with diabetes. Can you help me?

Most people who are told they have diabetes feel very upset at the news. We agree that a phone call to Diabetes UK helpline is a good idea; it has gone to a lot of trouble to produce useful information for people with newly diagnosed diabetes. However, the most important thing they can do is put you in touch with the local voluntary group of Diabetes UK. Naturally these vary in their level of activity, but in some areas are very well organised to provide support and information to new members. This will give you the opportunity to speak to other people who are in the same boat.

In the first few days, the nurse who showed you how to take insulin will give you the basic information you need to keep safe. Depending on how you get on, you will gradually take on board more complex information so that in time, you will be able to cope with any situation which might arise. It is essential to spend time with a dietitian who is experienced in diabetes because understanding the relationship between food and insulin is a key to good

MORECAMBE BAY HOSPITALS NHS TRUST

control. Once you have adjusted to life with diabetes, you should be offered an education programme, such as DAFNE (see p. 91).

DIET

Knowing about the right type of food and the amount that you can eat is important. Most of the questions we have included help explain the general principles but people's diets are very individual, so do ask for help and further explanations from your own diabetes advisor or dietitian. It is particularly important to have an opportunity to review regularly what you are doing about diet. If you are looking for new ideas for meals, there are now many helpful recipe books written especially for people with diabetes, most of which are available from Diabetes UK. A list of current titles can be found in Appendix 1.

I have had Type 1 diabetes for four years and am about to leave school. I don't eat a lot but cannot lose weight. Why is this?

Our bodies need energy from food and drink in order to function. Extra energy is required for any additional activity, such as walking, housework, climbing stairs or gardening. This energy is measured in calories or joules (see below).

To maintain a stable weight our energy intake (from food and drink) has to equal our energy output (for our daily activities.)

If your weight is increasing, your energy intake is exceeding your energy output, and the extra energy is stored as body fat. Even small differences in this balance will, in time, make a difference. An extra 100 calories (e.g. two small plain biscuits or one chocolate digestive) a day will amount to over 4.5 kg (over 10 lbs) weight gain in a year. Keeping a record of your food and drink intake can help you identify where you can make gradual changes, as your aim would be to reduce your food intake or increase your activity level, or ideally both.

In the UK we normally refer to calories, but some countries refer to joules: 1 calorie is equal to 4.2 joules. Strictly speaking, the proper term is kilocalories (often abbreviated to kCal) and kilojoules (abbreviated to kjoules or kJ). These are the units on the nutritional information labels on food packaging. Most people use the familiar term 'calorie' when they mean kilocalories, so this is what we have chosen to use in this book.

When you are taking insulin, it can be difficult to lose weight because unless you reduce your insulin at the same time as you cut back on food, you may be at risk of a hypo. The only way of correcting a hypo is to take extra carbohydrate, which defeats the object. You may need advice from your dietitian or specialist nurse on how to cut back on food and insulin.

There seem to be many foods offered in the supermarkets now labelled 'diabetic foods'. Should I be eating these rather than the ordinary types?

'Diabetic foods' do not offer any health benefits. They are expensive and are often no lower in fats or calories than ordinary food. They can still affect your blood glucose and can cause bowel upset.

In place of ordinary sugar these foods are sweetened with a substitute, often fructose or sorbitol, both of which provide calories and can have a laxative effect.

Today the recommended food plan for people with diabetes includes some sweetened foods, especially if you choose products with a higher fibre and lower fat content. Depending on your glucose control and your weight, you should be able to eat small amounts of ordinary sweet foods, such as biscuits, cakes or sweets but you may need to take extra insulin. These should form part of your food plan and should preferably be eaten at the end of a meal. There is no need for you to buy so-called diabetic foods to give yourself a treat.

The only 'special' foods we recommend for people with diabetes are the ones labelled as 'diet' or 'low calorie', e.g. sugar-free soft drinks, reduced sugar preserves, diet yoghurts and sugar-free jellies.

These are not marketed specifically at people with diabetes, but for anyone who wants to keep their weight under control or avoid eating too much sugar. They are usually sweetened with intense sweeteners such as saccharin or aspartame which are virtually calorie-free. These artificial sweeteners can also be used to replace sugar in your tea or coffee, and are available in granular form to sprinkle on break-fast cereal, or for use in baking.

Where or how do I find out about the carbohydrate or calorie content of foods?

There are many publications giving this information which are available in newsagents and bookshops. If you have access to the internet then a search will give you a great number of options. If you do not have access to the internet, your local library or Diabetes UK Careline may be able to help.

Another source of information is the nutritional labels on the foods you buy. If you find food labels difficult to understand then your dietitian will be able to explain how to use this information. The following tables give some examples of what you may see on labels.

People often ask for figures of how much to look for on a label and Table 2.3 can provide some *guidelines*. It must be noted that the figures are per 100 g of a food and each food choice should be taken in context of how much of it you eat and how often you eat it. No food needs to be excluded from an eating plan, but you should try to make sensible choices.

How does a person with diabetes get an appointment with a dietitian? Will there be one at my doctor's?

As diet plays a crucial part in the management of diabetes, it is important that you get sound expert dietary advice from a State Registered Dietitian. This is part of the recommended standard of care as detailed in the Diabetes UK booklet *What Diabetes Care to Expect* (see Appendix 1).

Table 2.1 General nutritional information on food labels

	TYPICAL VALUES		
	Per 100 g	Per serving 200 g	What this means
Energy	232 kJ 55 kCal	464 kJ 110 kCal	Energy or calories from this food. Limiting total calories will help you lose weight
Protein	4.5 g	9 g	For body growth and repair. Most adults get more than they need
Carbohydrate *of which sugars*	8.9 g 7.8 g	17.8 g 15.6 g	Total carbohydrate includes both starch and sugar. Both will affect blood glucose. Sugars include natural (fruit and milk) sugars and added sugar
Fat *of which saturates*	0.1 g 0.1 g	0.2 g 0.2 g	Three main types: monounsaturates, polyunsaturates, saturates; all contribute high energy. Aim to eat fewer fats – especially saturates
Fibre	0.1 g	0.2 g	Important for good bowel function
Sodium	0.1 g	0.2 g	High levels associated with high blood pressure

The availability of dietitians varies across the country but most diabetes centres have a dietitian as part of their diabetes team. If you attend a hospital diabetes centre then you should be able to make an appointment with the dietitian. There are an increasing number of GP practices running local diabetes clinics and they should be able to arrange an appointment with a dietitian as part of your diabetes care.

Table 2.2 Guideline Daily Amounts

Each day	Women	Men
Calories	Up to 2000	Up to 2500
Fat	Up to 70 g	Up to 95 g
Sugars	Up to 50 g	Up to 70 g
Salt	No more than 6 g	No more than 6 g

Table 2.3 Further guidance on food labels

This is *HIGH*	This is *LOW*
Per 100 g	Per 100 g
20 g fat or more	3 g fat or less
5 g saturated fat or more	1 g saturated fat or less
0.5 g sodium or more (multiply by 2.5 = salt)	0.1 g sodium (multiply by 2.5 = salt)
10 g sugar or more	2 g sugar or less

I have a number of queries about my diet. Can you tell me how I can get advice about it?

If you have access to the internet you might try the Diabetes UK website which provides a huge amount of information which may help answer your dietary queries (www.diabetes.org.uk). It also provides a telephone service called Diabetes Careline UK: 0845 120 2960.

Good advice on diet is essential in the proper care of diabetes and it should be tailored to individual requirements. You may therefore prefer to arrange to see a State Registered Dietitian through your hospital or your GP. Most hospitals have a State Registered Dietitian attached to the diabetes clinic, and you could arrange to see them at your next clinic visit. Some general practitioners organise their own diabetes clinics, and may arrange for a dietitian to visit this clinic. Many nurses and health visitors who are specially trained in diabetes will be able to provide basic dietary advice.

Do all alcoholic drinks affect my blood sugar level and if so, do they all have the same effect?

Alcoholic drinks contain varying amounts of alcohol and sugar, so different alcoholic drinks will have different effects on your blood glucose levels. They can be divided into those that contain sugar and those that do not. Sugar-containing drinks include beer, lager, cider, sweet sherry, port, Martini, alcopops such as Hooch and Bacardi Breezer, sweet dessert wine and liqueurs. The sugar content of these alcoholic drinks leads to an initial rise in the blood glucose level. The higher the sugar content, and the more of it you drink, the more your blood glucose will rise. Alcoholic drinks that do not contain sugar and therefore do not cause a rise in blood glucose include red and white wines, champagne, dry sherry and spirits such as whisky and gin. Examples of the sugar and calorie content of alcoholic drinks are given in Table 2.4.

The alcohol content of a drink has a separate effect on blood glucose levels and can cause delayed hypos; see the section *Alcohol* in Chapter 5.

I have had diabetes for 22 years and have only recently come back under the care of my local hospital. When I talked about my diet to the dietitian she was keen to make some changes, saying that there were quite a lot of new ideas and diet recommendations. What are these and is it worth me changing after all this time?

Dietary advice has certainly changed a lot since you were diag-nosed 22 years ago. As we learn more about food and how our bodies use it the advice about diet has to be adjusted. It is certainly

Table 2.4 Alcoholic drinks

Drink	Serving size	Units of alcohol	Calories kCal	Carbohydrate or sugar
Spirits, e.g. whisky, vodka, rum, gin	25 mL	1	52	trace
Spirits, e.g. whisky, vodka, rum, gin	35 ml	1.5	73	trace
Lager, 3.5–4.5% vol (e.g. Tennent's, Fosters)	pint	2.2	166	10 g
Lager, premium, Special Brew	pint	4.5	338	14 g
Lager, alcohol free, bottled	300 mL	Trace	21	4.5 g
Beer (bitter)	pint	2.2	184	13 g
Cider, dry	pint	2.7	206	15 g
Cider, sweet	pint	2.7	240	25 g
Wine, dry white or red, 12.5% vol	125 mL	1.6	112–120	trace
Wine, dry white or red, 12.5% vol	175 mL	2.2	157–168	trace
Wine, med. white, 12.5% vol	125 mL	1.6	120	4.3 g
Wine, sparkling, 10% vol	125 mLl	1.2	93	6 g
Sherry, dry, 20% vol	50 mL	1	58	trace
Sherry, med. 20 % vol	50 mL	1	58	3 g
Port	50 mL	1	79	6 g

worth knowing the new recommendations and it is never too late to make changes.

Dietary advice is now based on the principle of healthy eating which is encouraged for the population as a whole – not just for people with diabetes. The idea is that the whole family can be involved in good health rather than people with diabetes feeling they need a special diet. The major differences are an emphasis on:

- reducing fats, especially saturated fats;
- increasing fruit and vegetables.

There is now greater flexibility in choice: it is no longer forbidden to have sugar or sugary foods but advice is given on how much is recommended. In the last few years, stimulated by the introduction of the DAFNE programme (see p. 91), we now emphasise the relationship between carbohydrate and insulin. Carbohydrate counting is regarded as essential information for people with Type 1 diabetes as it allows them to adjust their insulin accurately for any food they want to eat. Lists of carbohydrate values are available from Diabetes UK.

So it is worth updating your diet. Your dietitian will provide individual advice, suited to your lifestyle. The main recommendations are summarised in Figure 2.1.

I am gradually losing my liking for sweet foods. When I do have them I follow my dietitian's advice and make sure that it is at a time when they are least likely to result in high blood glucose. However, I really do not enjoy my selection of high-fibre breakfast cereals without some sweetener – I was a Sugar Puff fan before! Can I put a little sugar on?

It is quite all right for you to use a small amount of sugar on your breakfast cereal if you wish. The current dietary recommendations for diabetes recognises that up to 10% of your daily energy intake may be taken as sucrose provided that it is in the context of a healthy diet. However, if you would prefer to 'save' sugar for some other food, or to 'save' calories, then using an artificial sweetener would be the best alternative.

There are many artificial sweeteners on the market, both in tablet and granular forms. It's just a matter of taste what you choose. The tablet form of the intense sweeteners is calorie and carbohydrate free. The granular forms have a small amount of carbohydrate but because the product is so light and the portion serving is so small this will not have any significant effect on your blood glucose. Many supermarkets have their own brand names but some examples are Canderel, Sweetex, Shapers, Splenda and Hermesetas.

Figure 2.1 Guidelines for healthy eating for diabetes

GUIDELINES FOR HEALTHY EATING FOR DIABETES

- Have regular meals – which include starchy carbohydrate foods such as bread, potatoes, rice, pasta, chapattis, cereals. We encourage high-fibre starchy foods and foods with a lower glycaemic index (see Table 3.3).

- Cut down on fats – especially saturated (animal) and hydrogenated fats – trans fatty acids (found in some margarines, manufactured cakes and biscuits), both linked to heart disease. Use less butter, margarine, cheese, cream and fatty meats. Grill, bake or steam rather than fry. Trim fat from meat, skin from chicken and skim fat from stews and stock. Include oily fish e.g. salmon, sardines, mackerel containing Omega 3 fat which may benefit health. Choose lower fat dairy products e.g. low-fat milk, low-fat or diet yoghurt. If using oil, choose monounsaturated e.g. olive or rapeseed oil. Remember to limit hidden sources of fat such as pies, pastries, cakes and biscuits.

- Fruit and vegetables – aim for at least five portions each day – e.g. 3 vegetables and 2 fruits. These provide vitamins and fibre, are low in fat and calories. A typical portion would be 3 tablespoons of vegetables, 1 apple, 1 orange, 1 pear, 2 kiwis, 2 satsumas, 2 plums, small handful of grapes, 1 small banana.

- Reduce sugar and sugary foods. This does not mean avoiding sugar. A small amount of sugar in foods or in baking as part of a healthy food plan is acceptable. Choosing sugar free and low sugar drinks is recommended.

- Reduce added salt. A high salt intake can increase blood pressure, so avoid added extra at the table, reduce amount in cooking and limit high salt foods like cheese, bacon, salted snacks. Herbs and spices are a good alternative flavouring. A gradual reduction in salt is often the most acceptable approach.
- Limit your intake of alcohol. The recommended intake is 3 units of alcohol for women and 4 units for men (see Table 2.4 for units of alcohol). Alcohol is a source of calories. Try to choose sugar-free mixers. Alcohol increases your risk of low blood glucose, so it is sensible never to drink on an empty stomach.
- Aim for weight control. If you are overweight, losing weight will help with the control of diabetes and reduce other risks such as heart disease and high blood pressure. Reducing weight gradually and increasing activity is encouraged. Even a small amount of weight loss is beneficial. Waist size is an important indicator for health risk (see Table 2.5).
- We do not recommend diabetic foods such as 'diabetic' biscuits and sweets as they have no health benefits. They are expensive, can affect your blood glucose, are a source of calories and can cause an unpleasant laxative effect.

Table 2.5 Definition of central obesity

Population group	Waist measurement
Caucasian (white) male	102 cm (40 inches)
Caucasian female	88 cm (35 inches)
Asian male*	88 cm (35 inches)
Asian female*	80 cm (32 inches)

*Asian people have a higher risk than Caucasians so the waist measurement is lower.

As a single parent I really find it hard to make ends meet. I know that very often I do not buy the foods that I should to help control my diabetes. Is there any way I can eat healthily but cheaply?

The food plan advised for people with diabetes should not cost more than the foods most people are eating before diagnosis. Having said that, when people have limited incomes, the amount available to spend on food makes it more difficult and challenging to have a healthy diet. The following tips may help, and you could also ask your dietitian for some more ideas.

Planning meals ahead and making a shopping list will help you not to buy on impulse. Avoid shopping when you are hungry as you are more likely to buy items not on your list. Supermarket own brands are often much cheaper. Bread is often sold for less near closing time. (Avoid buying bargains if you cannot store them.) Bread, pasta, rice, crackers and porridge are cheaper sources of energy than sugary foods and are much healthier. Frozen vegetables can be cheaper and easier to use, as long as you have a freezer.

Fruit may look expensive but not when you compare it to cakes, biscuits and sweets. If you can get to a market the fruit and vegetables there can be cheaper.

- **Breakfast** Try porridge, which is healthy and cheap and excellent for diabetes control. When it's too hot for porridge, try muesli: supermarket own brand or make your own from rolled oats, nuts and a little dried fruit, or supermarket own brand high-fibre cereal.

- **Lunch** A sandwich lunch can be very healthy, especially if you can use higher fibre, granary or pitta bread. Tinned sardines, mackerel or tuna are healthy, cheap choices for sandwich fillings. Tinned fish, scrambled egg or beans on toast can also be inexpensive. Homemade soups with added pulses (e.g. lentils) are filling and are a good source of protein and fibre.

- **Main meal** You do not need large helpings of meat at your main meal, and you can often extend it by adding tinned tomatoes or other tinned, frozen or fresh vegetables or adding pulses, e.g. beans and lentils. Diet yoghurts make excellent desserts and are good value for money. Another quick and healthy homemade dessert is a sugar-free jelly (available from most supermarkets), made up with milk or yoghurt, with fresh or tinned fruit.

The dietitian says that my high blood glucose levels during the morning may be caused by the pure fruit juice that I drink at breakfast. It is unsweetened juice, so how can this happen?

All fruit contains natural sugar and unsweetened fruit juices are no different. 'Unsweetened' means that the manufacturers have not added any extra sugar to the product. Many fruit juices are made from concentrated juice so can contain more sugar than the corresponding whole fruit. Juices are easy to drink and so your portion of fruit juice may be larger than you realise. Eating whole fruit is more limiting in quantity and because of the fibre content may produce a smaller effect on your blood glucose, but this is also dependent on the type of fruit or juice. It is acceptable to include fruit juice as part of a healthy diet but limiting the amount to a small glass at a time would be sensible. You can also dilute your fruit juice with mineral water or diet lemonade. You may prefer to choose a fruit juice with a lower carbohydrate/sugar content, e.g. tomato juice or 'light' cranberry juice (which uses artificial sweetener).

Overweight

I am trying to lose weight. How much should I lose a week?

It is best to lose weight gradually. If you are overweight then weight loss is to be encouraged but it is also important to keep the weight off. As you get used to the changes in your eating habits your new routine should become more familiar to you and make it less likely for you to lapse back to your old habits. Remember that if you are eating less carbohydrate, you will need to reduce your insulin doses. You may need to test your blood more frequently while you are getting used to the new diet.

A target loss of 0.5–1 kg (1–2 lb) per week is realistic and achievable for most people. Losing weight more rapidly can cause you to lose valuable muscle as well as fat. To lose 0.5 kg (1 lb) a week you have to reduce your calorie intake by 3500 calories per week (500 calories each day). Increasing your activity will also help to use up some of these calories. You may find that you lose more in one week and less in another, but this is quite normal as your body adjusts to your new plan. It is important not to give up at these times and continue to maintain your efforts. By keeping a food diary and looking carefully at your choices and portions of food you can make your own aims for change. Even a small amount of weight loss (5–10%) is known to improve control of diabetes, decrease blood pressure and improve blood fats (e.g. cholesterol). Remember that if you are cutting down on your carbohydrate intake, you will need to reduce your insulin to avoid the risk of hypos.

Fad diets may offer a quick fix but they are often unhealthy and most people find they cannot sustain them. It is common for people who lose weight too quickly to regain their previous weight *and more* within a few years.

Why are both my dietitian and diabetes specialist nurse so against my family buying me diabetic foods? I find my diet very hard to keep to and never lose weight anyway. So why can't I have diabetic foods as a treat?

Your dietitian and diabetes specialist nurse are not recommending the use of diabetic foods because those foods do not offer any health benefits. They are expensive and may affect your blood glucose. They are often high in fats and calories so will not help you lose weight. Finally they can produce an unpleasant laxative effect.

Having to follow any 'diet' is never easy and many people get fed up and find it hard to avoid what they perceive as forbidden foods.

There are no forbidden foods for people with diabetes but we do recommend sensible guidelines. Having an occasional treat is perfectly acceptable but it is important to recognise *how often* you have a treat and *how much* you have.

If you feel frustrated by not losing weight then a better goal for you may be weight maintenance. As we get older our weight normally increases so not gaining weight is still success.

I am very overweight and trying hard to lose about 20 kg (3 stone). I love ice-cream and most of the cheaper varieties in the supermarket contain non-milk fat. Will this be suitable for me?

You can choose to include a small bowl of ice-cream as part of your diet plan. Non-milk fat means that the manufacturers have used cheaper vegetable fats, which provide just as many calories as milk fat. Most ice-cream contains about 7–10% fat and around 80–120 calories per (2 oz/60 g) scoop – more in Cornish ice-cream. You can buy reduced calorie ice-cream but it is more expensive and you would have to decide if the saving in calories justified the cost. Like many foods it is helpful to identify how often and how much you eat them and aim to reduce the quantities and frequency in your efforts to reduce weight.

I have heard that there is a new appetite suppressant on the market but is it suitable for people with diabetes?

There are now two appetite suppressants which have been approved for use in diabetes. Both must be used in conjunction with a calorie reduced diet in order to achieve the desired weight loss.

- The most recent drug is rimonabant (Acomplia®) which works directly on the urge or craving to eat more. It appears to have relatively few side effects, but can cause depression. It is not recommended for people who have suffered from depression in the past.

- Sibutramine (Reductil®) has been on the market for some time and may be given to people with diabetes, who are above a certain weight (BMI 27 or higher). Sibutramine is not suitable for everyone and should not be used by people with heart disease. It can increase blood pressure so regular checks are necessary. Weight must be carefully monitored and the medicine discontinued if you have not lost 5% of your body weight in the first three months. It is not a long-term treatment and should not be taken for more than a year.

Although not an appetite suppressant, a further drug suitable for use in diabetes is orlistat (Xenical®). This works in the stomach and small intestine where it stops some of the fat from food being digested. This loss of fat is a loss of calories and therefore can aid weight loss. It is important that a low fat diet is followed to reduce unpleasant side effects. If you try this method of weight reduction, it is most important that you make use of the telephone helpline provided by the company. This comes with a package to help you make changes in your lifestyle.

I have the greatest difficulty losing weight and a friend has suggested that I should try joining Weight Watchers. Will they accept people with diabetes?

Weight Watchers and other slimming clubs can be very helpful to people who are having trouble losing weight, and that includes people with diabetes. They may ask for a letter from your doctor to confirm approval. We frequently encourage people to join a slimming club, which are often very successful in helping with weight loss where other efforts have failed. They can also support you after you have reached your target weight and need to maintain your weight loss. Any club which helps you with your motivation is to be encouraged. Weight Watchers advisors will not be able to help you with any changes in your insulin dose to compensate for any reduction in carbohydrate intake. You can always ask you diabetes team for advice.

EXERCISE

I've heard that exercise is particularly valuable for people with diabetes – is this true? If so, I'm not the sporty type and have never found going to the gym has any appeal to me. What should I do?

Exercise is good for people with diabetes but does not have to involve sports, and you can usually find something to suit your lifestyle. The staff at your local fitness centre are specially trained to help you with this, and these centres are a good place to start. They will work out an exercise programme with you and show you how to improve your fitness.

If you don't want to join a fitness centre, here are some other suggestions.

- Walk whenever you can and avoid using the car.

- Climb stairs rather than take the lift.

- Walk to and from work.

- Take your dog for more or longer walks.

- Consider buying a bicycle or exercise bike.

- Make a point of taking at least three half-hour walks a week at a fast pace.

- Take up swimming.

Depending on the intensity and duration of the exercise, you will need to reduce your insulin dose or take extra carbohydrate. There is advice about how to cope with insulin and exercise in Chapter 5: **Life with diabetes**.

If I keep to a good diet, why do I need to exercise as well?

Regular exercise stimulates a series of events in the body that result in changes in body composition. It reduces the amount of fat and increases the amount of lean tissue: muscle, fibres and bone. This increases your metabolic rate and improves your fitness, which is the amount of exercise that you can do without getting tired or exhausted. This not only makes you feel better but also reduces blood pressure and the 'bad' cholesterol (low density, LDL) and increases the 'good' cholesterol (high density, HDL). (See the question below on cholesterol.) Increasing fitness also increases the body's sensitivity to insulin and lowers blood glucose levels. It may also increase the tendency to develop hypoglycaemia and you might be able to reduce your insulin dose as your fitness improves.

I have been for a cholesterol check-up, but I noted that the doctor also wanted to check for HDL and LDL. What's the difference between all these measurements and what are they?

Cholesterol is a fat (lipid) and an important normal component of many body tissues including hormones. Its concentration in the blood, where it circulates attached to a protein (hence it is called a 'lipoprotein'), has been shown to be a valuable indicator of the risk of developing vascular disease. High levels of cholesterol are associated with an increased risk of heart attacks. There are two major components of cholesterol: low density lipoprotein (LDL) and high density lipoprotein (HDL). LDL cholesterol is the major risk factor for heart disease and is sometimes called 'bad' cholesterol. HDL, on the other hand, is the 'good' cholesterol since high levels of HDL protect against heart disease. Thus a high total cholesterol value is ambiguous unless you know whether it is due to increased LDL or HDL. Since insulin causes a rise in HDL cholesterol, people with Type 1 diabetes may have a high level of this 'good' cholesterol. Before contemplating any treatment for high cholesterol, your doctor needs to know that it is the 'bad' cholesterol (LDL) that is to blame. It is a complicated story and we hope this explanation helps. Visit: www.lipidsonline.org for more information.

NON-MEDICAL TREATMENTS

Recently I saw a physical training expert demonstrating a technique for achieving complete relaxation. She concluded by saying 'Of course, this is not suitable for everyone, for example people with diabetes.' Is this true and, if so, why?

This sounds like an example of ignorant discrimination. There is no reason why people with diabetes should not practise complete relaxation if they want to. If the session went on for a long time, you might have to miss a snack or even a meal but as you are burning up so little energy in a relaxed state, it should not matter.

My back has troubled me for many years and a friend has suggested that as a last resort I should try acupuncture. Would there be any objection to this, given that I have diabetes? Might it even help my diabetes?

Acupuncture has been a standard form of medical treatment in China for 5000 years. In the last 20 years it has become more widely used in this country. In China acupuncture has always been thought of as a way of preventing disease and is considered less effective in treating illness. In the UK acupuncture tends to be used by people who have been ill (and usually in pain) for a long time. It is most often tried in such conditions as a painful back, where orthodox medicine has failed to help. Even practitioners of the art do not claim that acupuncture can cure diabetes, but it will not do it any harm either, provided that you do not alter your usual diabetes treatment while you are having your course of acupuncture. If you have neuropathy (see Chapter 9) and have little sensation, it may be sensible to avoid acupuncture in the affected areas.

Do you think that complementary or alternative medicine can help people with diabetes?

Alternative medicine suggests a form of treatment that is taken in the place of conventional medical treatment. As such this could potentially be very dangerous as you cannot live without insulin.

However, there may be a place for complementary therapies that can be tried alongside conventional medicine. Although there is no scientific evidence to show that complementary therapies such as yoga, reflexology, hypnosis or aromatherapy can benefit someone with diabetes, some people who have tried them report that they feel more relaxed. As stress can have a detrimental effect on blood glucose control, it may mean that their diabetes improves as a result.

You should not alter your recommended diet or stop taking your insulin. No reputable complementary practitioner would suggest that you do this.

I have heard that there are herbal remedies for diabetes. What would these be?

There are many plants that have been said to reduce the high level of blood glucose in people with diabetes. One of these is a berry from West Africa and another a tropical plant called karela or bitter gourd. Some people have told us that they need less insulin if they take bitter gourd but there are no herbal remedies for Type 1 diabetes.

I recently read an article on ginseng that said it was beneficial to people with diabetes. Have you any information on this?

Ginseng comes from Korea and the powdered root is said to have amazing properties. There is no scientific evidence to suggest that it is of any help to people with diabetes.

*My little girl has just contracted diabetes at the age of three.
I would do anything to cure her. Would hypnosis be worth a try?*

Most parents are desperate for a cure when their child develops diabetes. In one sense, insulin injections are a cure in that they replace the missing hormone, but this is not much consolation to a distressed parent. Although a sense of desperation is natural, it is best for your child's sake for you to try to accept that she will always have diabetes. In this way she is more likely to come to terms with the condition herself. It is normal to grieve but at some stage you must face facts as a family and make use of all the help that is available for you and your daughter. In that way she will be less upset about her diabetes than you are. Hypnosis will not help her insulin cells to regenerate.

*An evangelistic healing crusade claims to heal among other
diseases 'sugar diabetes', malignant growth and multiple
sclerosis, etc. Are these claims correct?*

There are, of course, a handful of (unproven) reports of miracle cures of various serious diseases like cancer, but these are few and far between. A mildly overweight person might be persuaded to lose weight by a faith healer and so it might appear that the diabetes was 'cured', but no person on insulin has ever benefited from a healing crusade except in the strictly spiritual sense.

3 | Treatment with insulin

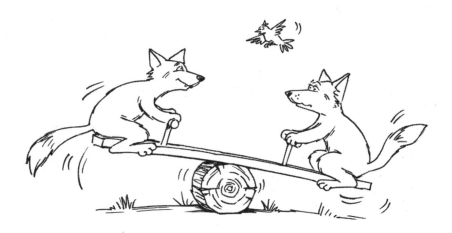

Insulin was discovered by Frederick Banting and Charles Best in the summer of 1921. The work was carried out in the Physiology Department of Toronto University while most of the staff were on their holidays. Before insulin was discovered, there was no treatment for people with diabetes and death inevitably occurred, usually within a year of diagnosis. The first human to be given insulin was a 14-year-old boy named Leonard Thompson who was dying of diabetes in Toronto General Hospital. This was an historic event, representing the beginning of modern treatment for diabetes. It was then up to the chemists to transform the production of insulin into an industrial process on a vast scale.

When Dr Robin Lawrence heard the news, he was in Florence waiting to die from diabetes. He drove straight to King's College

Hospital and arrived 'more dead than alive'. Three days later he received 20 units of insulin at 10 a.m. – by 4 p.m. he had his first hypo. He lived on and set up the first diabetic clinic in the UK. With the author HG Wells, he went on to found the British Diabetic Association, now called Diabetes UK.

Insulin has to be given by injection because at present it is inactivated if taken by mouth. Inhaled insulin has just been released but it not available for general use in the UK (see question on inhaled insulin, p. 43). About a quarter of all people with diabetes are treated with insulin. Virtually everyone who develops diabetes when they are young needs insulin from the time of diagnosis. People diagnosed in later life may manage quite satisfactorily for many years on other forms of treatment but eventually many of them will need insulin to supplement the diminishing supply of insulin from their pancreas.

People on insulin still have to take account of what they eat. There is a section *Diet and insulin* in this chapter, but we suggest that you also read the section on *Diet* in Chapter 2. However, healthy eating is only part of the treatment. Being the right weight and getting enough exercise is also important. There is a section *Sports* in Chapter 5 we suggest you look at.

The section *Hypos* (low blood glucose) is one of the most important parts of this book. It is the fear of hypos that prevents some people from controlling their blood glucose tightly. Diabetes care teams are often criticised for not giving people who are newly diagnosed enough information on hypos. So if you have just started insulin treatment, read this section carefully.

TYPES OF INSULIN

Since the discovery of insulin, countless people with diabetes have injected themselves with insulin extracted from the pancreas of cows and pigs. In the last 20 years or so human insulin has become widely available. However, human insulin is not extracted from human pancreas in the same way beef or pork insulin is. A great deal of research went into producing 'human' insulin by means of genetic engineering. This means that the genetic material of a bacterium or a yeast is reprogrammed to make insulin instead of the proteins it would normally produce. The insulin manufactured in this way is rigorously purified and contains no trace of the original bacterium.

The first insulin to be made was clear soluble insulin also called short-acting insulin. Injected under the skin, this insulin works within about 30 minutes and lasts for 4–8 hours. Various modifications were made to this original insulin so that it would last longer after injection. When protamine or zinc is incorporated into the soluble insulin, a single injection could last from 12 to 36 hours. For many years a single daily injection was advised by doctors, but people realised that this was not a good way of controlling the variations in blood glucose that occur during the day. Nowadays many people who need insulin have a mixture of short- and intermediate- or long-acting insulin twice a day, but an increasing number have insulin four or more times a day, injected using an insulin pen (see the section *Insulin pens* later in this chapter). A new generation of insulins, also called insulin analogues, where the chemical make-up of the insulin is changed, are also available today. By changing the molecular structure of the insulin, manufacturers can alter the way it works, allowing it to be absorbed differently.

I have heard that human insulin may be dangerous. There was a television programme which described many problems caused by human insulin. I have been taking human insulin for five years and am worried that it could have done me harm.

When human insulin was first introduced in 1982, many people were changed from insulin extracted from cattle or pigs to human insulin with the feeling that it would do them good. Many people were given little information about changes they might notice in the way the new insulin worked. All the experiments carried out by the insulin manufacturers before they launched human insulin suggested that it would work in exactly the same way as animal-derived insulin. Most people got on well with the new insulin but some people reacted very badly to it. They found that the warning of hypos was different and in a few cases that they felt extremely unwell while taking human insulin. They were transferred to their prior animal insulin and felt fine again. People like you, who were started on human insulin from the beginning, have no reason to fear bad reactions to this insulin.

A self-help group exists for people who are treated with insulin. The Insulin Dependent Diabetes Trust has highlighted a number of problems connected with insulin and the delivery of care. It has been an effective pressure group over the question of human insulin. See Appendix 2 for details.

My diabetes has been well controlled on beef insulin (soluble and isophane) for the past 32 years. Should I use human insulin instead?

Provided that you are doing well on your present insulin, there is no need to change. Although the major insulin companies have not made beef insulin for many years, a firm called CP Pharmaceuticals supplies beef and pork insulin under the brand names Hypurin® Bovine and Hypurin® Porcine. They produce:

- short-acting insulin: Hypurin Bovine Neutral and Hypurin Porcine Neutral;

- intermediate-acting insulin: Hypurin Bovine Isophane and Hypurin Porcine Isophane;

- long-acting insulin: Hypurin Bovine.

I have been taking beef insulin for many years and am worried about the possibility of this insulin being contaminated with BSE. Is this possible?

The manufacturers of beef insulin consider that the risk of any BSE (bovine spongiform encephalopathy) agent remaining after the intensive purification processes used to extract insulin is either negligible or non-existent. In addition, beef insulin used in the UK is derived from cattle originating in countries with a negligible incidence of BSE, so that the risk of coming into contact with BSE through beef insulin is very small indeed.

I have seen a programme on television, which says that human insulin may be dangerous. My 14-year-old son has just developed diabetes and I see that the doctor has put him on human insulin. You can imagine how worried I am about it.

Yes, it is unfortunate that this programme appeared at such a bad time for you. The people who make these programmes do not realise the fear and anxiety that they can cause.

First you must believe that your son needs insulin – without it he would soon become very ill. It does not really matter at this stage what sort of insulin he has, although most doctors start people who need insulin on the human variety. The only problems with human insulin seem to be caused by the changeover from animal to human insulin. As your son has been on human insulin or an analogue from the start, he should not run into any difficulties. Perhaps you should talk to a family with a child who has had diabetes for a few years. They would probably be able to give the reassurance you need. You could try contacting the local Diabetes UK voluntary group. They should be able to tell you if there is a local parents' group, or put you in touch with the family of a child with diabetes.

I have recently heard that human insulin can be dangerous, although I've taken it for several years. Should I be worried?

There has been adverse publicity about human insulin, which has been mentioned in the preceding questions. A number of people changing from animal to human insulin have noticed that they get less warning of hypos. This change of awareness may result from other factors (see the section *Hypos* later in this chapter) but some people are convinced that the problem was caused by human insulin.

There have also been reports of unexpected deaths in people who have changed to human insulin. These deaths may have been due to a low blood glucose but this has not been proved. Nor has it been shown that the numbers involved have increased since human insulin was introduced. Diabetes UK has been carrying out research into these vital questions but so far no cause for alarm has been found.

I am a Muslim and have been put on insulin. I hear that this is made from pork. Is this right?

Yes and no. Some insulins are pork-based, and there are pork-based synthetic insulins, both of which are unacceptable to Muslims. You need to inform your doctor or nurse of your wishes, stating that you wish to use a non-porcine synthetic (human) insulin instead. 'Human insulin' is not manufactured from human tissue, but is so called because it is 'akin to human'.

I've had diabetes for ten years and still hate giving insulin injections. I hear that at last inhaled insulin is available. How do I get hold of it?

Inhaled insulin (Exubera®) sounds like the answer to many people's prayers. However, it is by no means a universal solution to the need for insulin injections. In the first place the equipment needed to deliver

Table 3.1 Insulins available in the UK (August 2006)

Rapid-acting (analogue) insulin which is clear, has an onset of action within 15 minutes, a peak action of 30–70 minutes and lasts 2–5 hours

Name	Manufacturer	Source	Vial or cartridge[a]	Prefilled pen
Humalog	Lilly	Analogue	Cartridge and vial	Humalog Pen
NovoRapid	Novo Nordisk	Analogue	Cartridge	Flexpen
Apidra	Sanofi-Aventis	Human	Cartridge and vial	Optiset Pen

Soluble insulin which is clear, has an onset of action around 30 minutes, a peak action of 2–3 hours and lasts for 4–6 hours

Name	Manufacturer	Source	Vial or cartridge	Prefilled pen
Humulin S (Soluble)	Lilly	Human	Cartridge and vial	No
Insuman Rapid	Sanofi-Aventis	Human	Cartridge	Optiset Pen
Actrapid	Novo Nordisk	Human	Vial	No
Hypurin Porcine Neutral[†]	Wockhardt UK	Pork	Cartridge and vial	No
Hypurin Bovine Neutral[†]	Wockhardt UK	Beef	Cartridge and vial	No
Porcine Actrapid (until Dec. 2007)	Novo Nordisk	Pork	Cartridge and vial	No
Velosulin (until Dec. 2007)	Novo Nordisk	Human	Vial	No

Intermediate acting insulin which is cloudy and lasts 6–24 hours with a peak action of 4–8 hours

Name	Manufacturer	Source	Vial or cartridge	Prefilled pen
Humulin I (isophane)	Lilly	Human	Vial and cartridge	Humulin I Pen
Insulatard	Novo Nordisk	Human	Vial and cartridge	Innolet
Insuman Basal	Sanofi-Aventis	Human	Vial and cartridge	Optiset Pen
Porcine Insulatard (until Dec. 2007)	Novo Nordisk	Pork	Vial	No
Hypurin Porcine Isophane†	Wockhardt UK	Pork	Vial and cartridge	No
Hypurin Bovine Isophane†	Wockhardt UK	Beef	Vial and cartridge	No

Intermediate/Long-acting analogue insulin which is clear and lasts between 12 and 24 hours with no peak action

Name	Manufacturer	Source	Vial or cartridge	Prefilled pen
Levemir (detemir)	Novo Nordisk	Analogue	Cartridge	Flexpen
Lantus (glargine)	Sanofi-Aventis	Analogue	Vial and cartridge	Optiset Pen

ªVials are bottles of insulin for use with a syringe, and cartridges are for use with an insulin pen

Table 3.1 Insulins available in the UK (August 2006) *continued*

Long-acting insulin

Name	Manufacturer	Source	Vial or cartridge	Prefilled pen
Hypurin Bovine Lente[†]	Wockhardt UK	Beef	Vial	No
Hypurin Bovine PZI[†]	Wockhardt UK	Beef	Vial	No

Mixed insulin containing short-acting and intermediate-acting insulin in varying proportions

Name	Manufacturer	Source	Vial or cartridge	Prefilled pen
Mixtard 10 (until Dec. 2007)	NovoNordisk	Human	Cartridge	No
Mixtard 20 (until Dec. 2007)	NovoNordisk	Human	Cartridge	No
Mixtard 30	NovoNordisk	Human	Cartridge	Innolet
Mixtard 40 (until Dec. 2007)	NovoNordisk	Human	Cartridge	No
Mixtard 50 (until Dec. 2007)	NovoNordisk	Human	Cartridge	No
Humulin M3	Lilly	Human	Vial and cartridge	Humulin M3 Pen
Insuman Comb 15	Sanofi-Aventis	Human	No	Optiset Pen
Insuman Comb 25	Sanofi-Aventis	Human	Vial and cartridge	Optiset Pen
Insuman Comb 50	Sanofi-Aventis	Human	Cartridge	Optiset Pen
Porcine Mixtard 30 (until Dec. 2007)	NovoNordisk	Pork	Vial	No
Hypurin Porcine Mix 30/70[†]	Wockhardt UK	Pork	Vial and cartridge	No

Mixed insulin comprising rapid-acting analogue insulin and intermediate-acting analogue insulin

Name	Manufacturer	Source	Vial or cartridge	Prefilled pen
Humalog Mix 25** Pen	Lilly	Analogue	Cartridge	Humalog Mix 25
Humalog Mix 50** Pen	Lilly	Analogue	Cartridge	Humalog Mix 50
Novomix 30¶	Novo Nordisk	Analogue	Cartridge	Flexpen

#Vials are bottles of insulin for use with a syringe, and cartridges are for use with an insulin pen.

† All Hypurin packaging is marked with braille

* The numbers refer to the percentage of soluble (short-acting) to isophane (intermediate-acting) insulin, e.g. Humulin M3 is 30% soluble to 70% isophane

** Humalog mixes are a mixture of lispro solution and lispro protamine suspension (both analogue insulins)

¶ NovoMix 30 is 30% soluble insulin aspart and 70% insulin aspart protamine the insulin into your lungs is quite bulky and much larger than a simple inhaler for asthma. Secondly, the amount of insulin you would need to take into your lungs is ten times greater than you would give by injection and coupled with this is the extra cost, which is about twice that of injected insulin. Because the lungs are not designed to take in a large protein three or more times a day, there is a theoretical risk of lung damage, which could be a serious problem. Thus the manufacturers of inhaled insulin recommend that people taking this form of insulin should have tests on their lungs. They should be tested before starting this treatment, after six months, and then every year. It should not be used in people with asthma or lung disease. Smokers should not use Exubera till they have quit for six months. At present, Exubera is not routinely available in the UK as it has not been approved by NICE (see the next question).

I have heard to my amazement that although inhaled insulin is now available, it has not been approved by the licensing bodies in the UK. Can you please explain how people in need of insulin will be deprived of this new development?

In the UK, new medicines (including insulins) have to be passed by a body called the National Institute for Clinical Excellence, or NICE for short. This organisation examines each new medication and carries out a cost–benefit analysis to decide if it should be available on prescription from the NHS. In the case of people with diabetes, this means that it will be available at no cost, since they are bound to be exempt from prescription charges. NICE has been fairly resistant to the introduction of Exubera. We quote their recommendation in full.

> Inhaled insulin is not recommended for the routine treatment of people with Type 1 or Type 2 diabetes mellitus.
> Inhaled insulin may be used as a treatment option for people with Type 1 or Type 2 diabetes mellitus who show evidence of poor glycaemic control despite other therapeutic interventions (including, where appropriate, diet, oral hypoglycaemic agents [OHAs] and subcutaneous

insulin) and adequate educational support, and who are unable to initiate or intensify pre-prandial subcutaneous insulin therapy because of either:

- a marked and persistent fear of injections that meet DSM-IV criteria for specific phobia 'blood injection injury type' diagnosed by a diabetes specialist or mental health professional

- severe and persistent problems with injection sites (for example, as a consequence of lipohypertrophy) despite support with injection site rotation.

In patients receiving inhaled insulin under the circumstances set out above, treatment should only be continued beyond six months, and in the longer term, if there is evidence of a sustained improvement in glycated haemoglobin (HbA_{1c}) that is judged to be clinically relevant to the individual patient's overall risk of developing long-term complications of diabetes.

Initiation of inhaled insulin treatment and monitoring of response should be carried out only by a specialist centre.

There seem to be a lot of different types of insulin on the market. Can you give me some details?

The range of insulins available can be confusing, although they do fall into four separate groups which are shown in Table 3.1. The times of insulin action vary greatly from one person to another and those given must only be regarded as a rough guide.

The vials mentioned in the table are bottles of insulin for use with a syringe, and cartridges are for use with an insulin pen.

I am taking a mixture of short- and intermediate-acting insulin twice a day and do not understand which insulin is working at which time of day.

Many people are confused by the length of action of their insulin particularly when taken more than twice a day. The diagram in

Figure 3.1 gives a representation of some commonly used regimens. However, as a general rule the short-acting insulin works rapidly (morning and evening) and the intermediate-acting insulin takes longer and covers the afternoon and the night. If you are still unclear about it have another word with your doctor or diabetes specialist nurse.

Can I get AIDS from human insulin?

Definitely not. Human insulin is made either from bacteria or yeast 'instructed' to produce insulin that has the same structure as human insulin, or from pork insulin modified to resemble human insulin. It is rigorously purified and cannot be a source of infection.

Is it possible to be allergic to insulin?

Very occasionally people may develop an allergy to one of the additives to insulin such as protamine or zinc, but the insulin itself is unlikely to cause an allergy.

My doctor wants me to change to four injections a day. Is this necessary?

More and more people are taking four injections a day and in general they are happy with this arrangement, even though it obviously means more injections. Twice-daily insulin is a compromise with each injection containing a mixture of short- and long-acting insulin in the hope that this will provide the correct amount of insulin for each meal and the times in between eating.

We all need a small amount of insulin to trickle into our body throughout the day to keep our glucose level steady. We sometimes call this background (or basal) insulin and for people who are of a normal weight, this usually amounts to up to 24 units a day. The amount of background insulin needed varies under different circumstances, such as exercise, illness and after drinking alcohol, to name but a few. On top of this background insulin, we also need insulin with every meal (bolus insulin) to deal with the effects of food on the blood glucose. The actual amount of insulin needed depends on the type of food and in particular the amount of carbohydrate eaten. Many diabetes centres run courses to teach people how to match their insulin to carbohydrates. DAFNE is an example of such a course. See p. 51 for more about DAFNE.

Would I be able to achieve better control if I went onto three injections a day?

If you are on two insulin injections a day, you probably take a pre-mixed insulin such as Mixtard before breakfast and before your evening meal. It is possible to achieve good control with this sort of insulin, but many people find that they are unable to keep their sugar down at a certain time of day without running the risk of hypos at another time. This is a built-in problem with fixed mixtures of insulin. Most commonly, blood glucose is high at bedtime after a good evening meal. If this is the case, we suggest 'splitting the evening dose' of insulin by having short-acting insulin before your evening meal and long-acting insulin at bedtime. This will allow you to adjust the dose of each insulin to achieve good results without going hypo in the night.

I have heard people refer to 'basal bolus' insulin. What does this mean and is it effective?

Basal insulin is needed to maintain normal blood glucose levels, when the body is in a basal or resting state. This varies depending on the time of day and may be affected by illness and other conditions. It is normally given in the form of a long-acting insulin at night, which should last for 24 hours. If it fails to achieve this, another dose of long-acting insulin can be given in the morning. The word bolus comes from the Latin, meaning a cast of the dice or a lump: this refers to the insulin given before you eat to control the

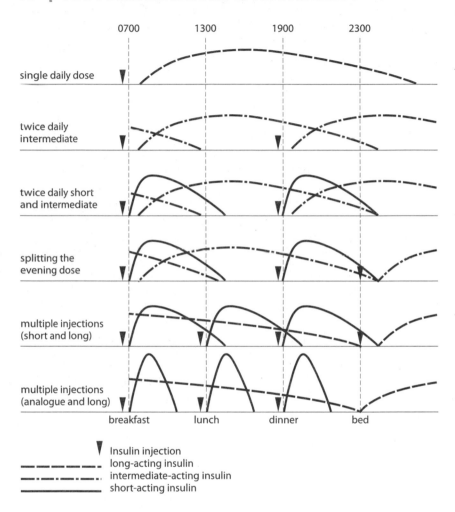

Figure 3.1 Five common insulin regimens

effect of food you are about to take in. This is normally a short-acting insulin or a rapid-acting analogue. This combination is now widely used in Type 1 and Type 2 diabetes and gives people the greatest flexibility in what they eat and when they eat it.

TIMING

I have heard that there is a new fast-acting insulin which is even faster-acting than Actrapid. Does it have any advantages?

You are quite right, there are now five new synthetic 'designer' insulins: three rapid-acting insulins – lispro (Humalog®), aspart (NovoRapid®) and Apidra® from Aventis. There are also two longer-acting versions: glargine (Lantus®) and detemir (Levemir®) They are the first of what will be a series of new insulins (known as insulin analogues) which will be produced in the years to come. They are designed so as not to aggregate when injected under the skin (a process that occurs to a varying extent with other insulins), thus speeding up their absorption and action. Their big potential advantage is – at least for Humalog and NovoRapid – that they don't need to be injected until immediately before the meal, and their action more closely matches the digestion of the meal than that of conventional clear insulins. This results in better control of the rise in blood glucose following meal digestion and absorption with lowering of the peak glucose concentration. They have another advantage, stemming from their short action: when injected before breakfast, they are less likely to cause hypos before lunch as their effects wear off more quickly. They are ideally suited for the popular 'basal plus bolus' regimens, that is, a long-acting 'basal' insulin at night with a 'bolus' of short-acting insulin before each meal, and are available in cartridges and disposable pens.

I have been having hypos at night and my doctor is keen to change my background insulin to a new long-acting insulin, which he says will solve the problem. How will this help?

He would probably like you to try one of the new insulin analogues. These last longer than your present insulin which is likely to be a form of isophane insulin. This was developed in

Denmark 60 years ago and has been the standard background insulin for the past 20 years. Isophane has the drawback that it only lasts for 12 to 16 hours and has a very variable absorption pattern. This means that even if you take identical doses of isophane on consecutive nights, the rate of absorption may vary greatly. This explains why you can wake with a glucose level of 7 one morning and 17 the next. The two new long-acting insulins have been designed to enter the bloodstream slowly and to last for up to 24 hours. Lantus® (glargine) probably has the longer action and lasts for 24 hours in many people. Levemir® (detemir) probably has a shorter duration of action than Lantus, but is said to have a more consistent action than other long-acting insulins. Most people who change from isophane to Lantus or Levemir get on well with the new insulin and find that their dose of background insulin is more effective and predictable.

My practice nurse would like me to try a new long-acting insulin but tells me there are two options and she is not sure which one to use in my case. Could you please elaborate?

There are two long-acting analogue insulins: detemir (Levemir®) and glargine (Lantus®). They are both 'designer' insulins which are intended to last for up to 24 hours. There is not much to choose between them. Detemir is probably more consistent in its action and glargine has a slightly longer duration of action. This means that as a background insulin, you are more likely to have to take detemir twice a day – usually before breakfast and at bedtime. Glargine is in a slightly acid solution and some people complain that it stings a little when injected.

For the past four years, I have used Actrapid insulin before meals and Insulatard at bedtime. I've recently been changed to NovoRapid as mealtime insulin and I'm not very happy. My control has got worse and I seem to need much larger doses of NovoRapid compared with the dose of Actrapid. It is very disheartening as I was told the new insulin would make life easier.

This is a common problem with changing to NovoRapid and there is a simple explanation. It concerns the need for background insulin 24 hours a day. Actrapid is a longer-acting insulin than NovoRapid and usually lasts from one meal to the next. Thus Actrapid before a meal provides the surge of insulin for the meal but once you are back in the basal (unfed) state, the activity of Actrapid persists, acting as background insulin until your next insulin injection. This has the downside of putting you at risk of a hypo before your next meal and increasing the need for snacks between meals. NovoRapid (exactly like Humalog) is designed to act more rapidly and wear off sooner than Actrapid. The risk of hypo is reduced but now there are times between meals when you have no background insulin.

There are two solutions to this problem. One is to take an extra injection of Insulatard before breakfast. This would last throughout the day until your second injection of Insulatard at bedtime. The other option is to change to a longer-acting analogue such as glargine or detemir. These last for up to 24 hours, unlike Insulatard which only has a duration of 16 hours. Whoever replaced your Actrapid with NovoRapid should have predicted this need to change your background insulin.

What should I do if I suddenly realise I have missed an injection?

It is quite easy to forget to give yourself an injection or – even worse – to be unable to remember whether or not you have had your injection. If this happens you should measure your blood glucose level to help you decide what to do next.

MORECAMBE BAY HOSPITALS NHS TRUST

If your blood glucose is high (more than 10 mmol/L) you probably did forget your injection and you should have some short-acting insulin as soon as possible. The dose depends on how close you are to the next injection time. If your blood glucose is normal or low (7 mmol/L or less) you probably did have your injection even if you have forgotten doing it. It would be safest to check your blood glucose again before your next meal and, if it is high, to have an extra dose of short-acting insulin.

Does the timing of the injections matter? Can a person who is on two injections a day take them at 10 a.m. and 4 p.m.?

Unless you are taking Humalog or NovoRapid, which are very quick-acting insulins and should be taken just before a meal, it is best to have your insulin about 30 minutes before a meal, and we discuss this further in the next section *Diet and insulin*. If you have your main meals in the middle of the morning and in the afternoon, then you could try giving insulin at the times you suggest. You may find that an afternoon injection may not last the 18 hours until the next morning, which is why most people try to keep their two injections about 12 hours apart.

DOSAGE

When I was first diagnosed I was put on insulin, but now the dosage has been decreased. The doctor tells me I am in the 'honeymoon period' of diabetes. What does this mean?

People often need a reduction in their insulin dose soon after they start taking insulin for diabetes. This is due to partial recovery of the insulin-producing cells of the pancreas. During this period hypos are often a problem but, on the whole, it is easy to control the blood glucose. The 'honeymoon period' usually comes to a sudden end within a few months to a year, often when the person has a bad cold or suffers some other stress to the insulin-producing cells. However, the honeymoon period is a good thing and will improve your chances of successful long-term control of your diabetes.

When I developed diabetes I was started on insulin but kept having hypos, and three months ago I came off insulin. Why was I given it in the first place?

Presumably you were given insulin because your doctors thought you needed it. Most people under 40 years old who have ketones in their urine (see the section *Urine testing* in Chapter 4) are likely to need insulin and tend to be started on this without any delay. When insulin has been given for a week or so, it is quite common for people to be troubled by hypos, in which case the insulin has to be reduced. Sometimes even tiny doses of insulin cause hypos during this 'honeymoon period' (see the previous question) and the injections have to be stopped completely. The honeymoon period may occasionally last as long as a year.

I have had diabetes for nine months and attend the diabetes clinic every month to have my insulin dose adjusted. How long does it usually take before nurses get you balanced?

This is an interesting question as it assumes that it is up to professionals to balance your diabetes. Of course the doctors and nurses in the clinic must provide you with all the help and information that you need but, in the end, it is up to you to control your diabetes. Good control depends not just on the dose of insulin but the site you choose for your injections, the timing and type of food that you eat and the amount of exercise you take. These are things over which your doctor or nurse has no direct control. Most people begin to get their blood glucose under control in a few weeks.

Is my insulin requirement likely to vary at different times of the year because of the weather?

Several people have remarked that their dose of insulin needs to be altered in very hot weather: some need to give themselves more insulin and others less. This is probably because people react in different ways to a heatwave. There is a tendency to eat less and take less exercise in tropical conditions. However, because blood flow to the skin is increased in warm temperatures, this could speed up the absorption of the injected insulin and mean that a given dose will not last as long. Everyone is different and you will have to find out for yourself how hot weather affects your own blood glucose.

If my insulin requirements decrease over the years, does this mean that the pancreas has gradually started to produce more natural insulin than when I was younger?

No. It is most unlikely that after many years of diabetes your pancreas will start to produce natural insulin. However, this reduction in dose in older people is well recognised. It could be that you were having more insulin than you really needed in the past. Since the introduction of blood glucose measurement many people are found to be having too much insulin, or sometimes too much at one time of the day and not enough at another. Other possible explanations for older people needing less insulin are that they eat less food, they become thinner, they have a different exercise pattern, and there may be hormonal changes.

INJECTING

Insulin pumps

I have heard about insulin pumps for treating diabetes. Doctors in my own clinic never seem very keen on the idea. How do pumps work and are they a good form of treatment?

First, an explanation of why insulin pumps have been developed. People who do not have diabetes release a very small amount of insulin into the bloodstream throughout the day and over the night. This insulin prevents the liver from releasing its glucose stock into the bloodstream. Whenever the glucose level rises after a meal the pancreas immediately produces extra insulin to damp the level down. This is a simple feedback system designed to keep the level of blood glucose steady. Without the 'background' insulin in between meals, the level of blood glucose would steadily rise.

Insulin pumps are an attempt to copy this normal pattern. They consist of a slow motor driving a syringe or cartridge containing insulin, which is pumped down a fine-bore tube and needle. The needle is inserted under the skin and strapped in place. There is also a device for giving mealtime boosts of insulin. Modern pumps are about the size of a pager, and a microprocessor-based button allows a wide range of rate settings.

Many people successfully control their blood glucose with an insulin pump. However, because of the cost, they are only available on the NHS under certain well-defined circumstances and this depends on funding from your local Primary Care Trust. They require extra blood tests and adjustments in the dose of insulin, but they can be a good way of achieving tight control of diabetes in people with a high degree of commitment.

My diabetes is well controlled. Should I be thinking of buying a pump?

An insulin pump is probably not necessary if your diabetes is already well controlled. However, there are some advantages in being able to set your background insulin at the desired rate for every hour of the day and night. This is particularly valuable if you are prone to night hypos.

Currently approximately 0.1% of people with Type 1 diabetes in the UK use pumps, compared with about 5% in the USA, The Netherlands, Sweden, Germany and Norway. Nevertheless, pump therapy is not suitable for all people with diabetes. Discussions with healthcare professionals, pump users and manufacturers suggest that the people most suited to using pumps must be well motivated and willing to take control of their diabetes, have a good knowledge and understanding of their diabetes, and be prepared to test blood glucose levels at least four times a day and be able to act on those results.

NICE (National Institute for Clinical Excellence), the government body which assesses the value of new forms of treatment, has recommended that pumps should only be funded by the NHS in a specific situation, namely people with Type 1 diabetes, in whom multiple injections have failed to provide good control and who have a problem with 'disabling hypos'. Visit the website: www.nice.org.uk/page.TA057 for more information.

NICE also recommends that insulin pumps should only be provided to people with 'the commitment and competence to use the therapy effectively'. However, we know some people who do very few blood tests but still manage to keep themselves out of hospital by using a pump.

What are the main difficulties in using a pump for giving insulin?

The main problem with pumps is that, like all machines, they are capable of going wrong. One reason for the high cost of insulin pumps is the need to build a warning system into the design to alert the user to a mechanical fault. If the pump suddenly stops, the user will rapidly run out of insulin and develop ketoacidosis (see question on ketones on p. 112).

Some people have problems with skin infections at the site of the needle, which acts as a foreign body. The skin must be cleaned carefully before inserting the needle, which should be replaced every two days.

The main disadvantage of the pump for some people is that it has to be worn day and night and is a constant reminder of their diabetes, in contrast to the ordinary injections, which are over and done with rapidly.

How can I obtain an insulin pump?

You must first discuss the use of the pump with your diabetes specialist nurse. Pumps are available free on the NHS for people with Type 1 diabetes, who fulfil certain criteria (see the two previous questions). There are three manufacturers supplying pumps in the UK: Roche (previously called Disetronic), Medtronic and Animas. Each of these pump manufacturers supports the intensive education that is essential in the early stages of pump use. The provision of pumps is a competitive business and some centres understandably tend to favour a particular supplier. If you want more information on insulin pumps, look at the website: www.insulin-pumpers.org.uk; Diabetes UK also has useful information on insulin pumps on its website.

Insulin pens

What is an insulin pen, and what are the advantages of using one?

An insulin pen consists of a cartridge of insulin inside a case like a fountain pen which is used with a special disposable needle. After dialling the required number of units of insulin and inserting the needle into the skin, you press the plunger or button and the pen will release the correct dose of insulin. There are also pens which have insulin built in and these are known as prefilled pens, preloaded or disposable pens. All cartridges and prefilled pens now contain 300 units of insulin and are likely to last several days before needing to be changed. Available pens are listed in Table 3.2. In general the pens are only compatible with insulin cartridges from the same manufacturer.

The great advantage of insulin pens is that they are easier to use than syringe and needle and more convenient. It is simple to give an injection away from home, for example at work, in a restaurant or when travelling. If your eyesight is not good you may find the dial-a-dose clicking sound helps to reassure you that you have dialled up the correct dose. Some pens give a distinct click with each unit or two units dialled.

If you suffer from arthritis or nerve damage in your hands you are likelier to find a pen easier to use than drawing up insulin in a conventional syringe. All these pens rely on ordinary finger pressure for the injection, that is, they are not automatic injectors, but some may be easier than others. For example, the InnoLet® prefilled pen has been especially designed to have a distinctive click and needs mild finger pressure to inject the insulin.

If you find it difficult to inject your insulin because of fear of needles, but would like to use a pen, Novo Nordisk has introduced the PenMate® which hides the needle from view when the injection is given. The PenMate can be obtained on prescription.

Several makes of pen are available and your healthcare professional will show you the current models. Insulin pens are now available on prescription except for the OptiClik Pen which can be obtained from your nurse. In an urgent situation most pens are available from your hospital diabetic clinic. It may help to have two pens so one can be used as a back-up in case of breakage or loss.

Addresses for all the companies mentioned here can be found in Appendix 2.

Table 3.2 Insulin pens

Company	Pen name	Increments	Dosage range	Insulin used in pen	Reusable or prefilled
Owen Mumford	Autopen Classic	1 unit	1–21	Insulin from Lilly or Wockhardt	Reusable
	Autopen Classic	2 units	2–42	Insulin from Lilly or Wockhardt	Reusable
	Autopen 24	1 unit	1–21	Glargine insulin (Lantus®)	Reusable
	Autopen 24	2 units	2–42	Glargine insulin (Lantus®)	Reusable
Novo Nordisk	Novopen 3 Classic	1unit	1–70	Any Novo Nordisk insulin	Reusable
	Novopen 3 Fun	1 unit	1–70	Any Novo Nordisk insulin	Reusable
	Novopen Junior	½ unit	1–35	Any Novo Nordisk insulin	Reusable
	Innolet	1 unit	1–50	Mixtard® 30 and Insulatard	Prefilled
	Flexpen	1 unit	1–60	NovoRapid®, Levemir® and Novomix 30	Prefilled
Lilly	Humapen Luxura	1 unit	1–60	Any Lilly insulin	Reusable
	Humapen Ergo	1 unit	1–60	Any Lilly insulin	Reusable
	Lilly Prefilled Pen	1 unit	1–60	Humalog® Mix50, Humalog® Mix25, Humalog, Humulin I and Humulin M3®	Prefilled
Sanofi-Aventis	OptiClik	1unit	1–80	Glargine insulin (Lantus®)	Reusable
	Optiset	2 units	2–40	Glargine insulin (Lantus®)	Prefilled
	Optipen Pro	1 unit	1–60	Any Sanofi-Aventis insulin	Reusable

I have been using animal insulin with a syringe but would really prefer to use a pen. Is this possible?

People who use animal insulin can use either a syringe or a pen injection device. The animal insulins available in cartridge form are:

- Hypurin® porcine neutral;

- Hypurin porcine isophane;

- Hypurin porcine 30/70 mix;

- Hypurin bovine neutral;

- Hypurin bovine isophane.

These are all manufactured by Wockhardt UK. They are recommended for use with the Owen Mumford Autopens (see Table 3.2).

I have been told I need four injections a day. I am worried that I might get the insulins mixed up. What can I do to prevent this?

Many people now take three, four or five insulin injections a day and this will mean using two or even three different types of insulin. This is known as a 'basal bolus' or multiple injection regimen. The 'basal' insulin is the long-acting background insulin and the 'bolus' dose is taken when a meal or a large snack is eaten. Some people may take a fixed mixture of insulin in the morning, a fast-acting insulin with their evening meal and a background insulin at bedtime.

The idea of using a multiple injection regimen is to try to mimic the normal insulin secretion of the pancreas, by giving small doses of short-acting insulin to cover meals and a longer-acting insulin once a day to act as a background insulin. The insulin pen was originally developed to make it more convenient for people to inject four times a day. We agree that it can be confusing if you are taking two or three insulins but most pens are available in different colours to help distinguish the different insulins being used. If you are using prefilled pens, these are already colour-coded.

Some people whose lifestyle means they eat at irregular times find their diabetes much more manageable with a basal bolus regimen. There is more flexibility over the timing of meals, as the insulin is not taken until just before the meal is eaten. In practice some people may also need some long-acting insulin taken in the morning to 'top up' the evening background insulin but this will depend on the type of insulin used.

Injectors

My son has trouble giving himself injections and has asked me if he can use an injector. What type of injector should he use?

There are two devices currently available which might help your son overcome his aversion to injections. The first is the AutoJect 2® made by Owen Mumford and the second is the PenMate® made by Novo Nordisk.

Injectors work by pushing the needle very quickly through the skin, while hiding the needle from view. As well as offering fast needle penetration, the AutoJect 2 also automatically delivers the insulin at speed with a conventional syringe. It is obtainable from Owen Mumford (Medical Shop) (address in Appendix 2). This injector is not available on prescription. If your son uses a Novopen®, then the Novo Nordisk device called PenMate slips over the NovoPen 3, Demi or Junior and inserts the needle into the skin automatically, while hiding it from view. This can be obtained on prescription from your GP.

What is the 'jet' injector?

This is a needle-free injector, which works by penetrating the skin with insulin using very high pressure jets. It is not entirely painless and is fairly bulky. The recent model available in the UK

(MHI-500) has been superseded by a new model, SQ-PEN; see the website www.SQ-PEN.com for details.

Practical aspects of pens, needles, syringes and bottles

When I was discharged from hospital with newly-diagnosed diabetes I was given a pen device and a few disposable syringes and needles for my injections. How do I obtain more?

Pen devices, disposable insulin syringes and pen needles are available free on prescription. Your GP will supply you with a prescription for any make of insulin syringe and/or insulin pen needles that you choose, and they can then be obtained without charge from a chemist. Alternatively you can buy them at your own cost directly from the chemist without a prescription, or you can send for them by post from suppliers such as Owen Mumford (Medical Shop). Their address is in Appendix 2.

What is the best way of disposing of insulin syringes and needles?

There is a device available called the BD Safe-Clip® which cuts the needle off the top of a syringe or insulin pen and retains it in the device. Once the needle is clipped off, put the used syringe or pen needle hub into a rigid sealable container (available on prescription as a Sharps bin) along with your lancets and follow your local council guidelines for safe disposal of medical waste. Some local authorities provide special containers and a collection service for people who are treated with insulin; however, there is no national policy.

The BD Safe-Clip is available free on prescription from your GP.

I have heard that pen needles and disposable syringes can be reused. How many times can they be reused and how can they be kept clean in between injections?

While pen needles and disposable syringes are designed to be used only once, some people do reuse them. However, reusing needles causes them to become blunt, and they can bend very easily. The tiny point on the end can also break off and remain embedded in the flesh. Needles have a fine coating of lubricant so they glide in and out of the skin. Reusing them removes this lubricant and may cause a more painful injection. So there are many reasons to use each needle once only.

If you decide to reuse them make sure the protective cover is placed over the needle.

There is a bewildering array of syringes and needles on the market. Which are the best types to use?

In the UK we use three sizes of syringe. They are used with U100 insulin, which is the standard strength of insulin in the UK and most other countries, containing 100 units of insulin per 1 millilitre.

- The 0.5 mL syringe. This is marked with 50 single divisions for taking not more than 50 units of insulin in one injection.

- The 1 mL syringe, marked up to 100 units in 2 unit divisions for those taking more than 50 units of insulin in one injection.

- The 0.3 mL syringe, designed for children or those taking less than 30 units of insulin in one injection.

The most popular make is the BD syringe which comes complete with a fixed Micro-Fine+ 12.7 mm needle, but there are several other makes available.

All these syringes are marked with the word INSULIN on the side of the syringe and graduated in units of insulin. No other type should be used to inject insulin. They are all shown in Figure 3.2.

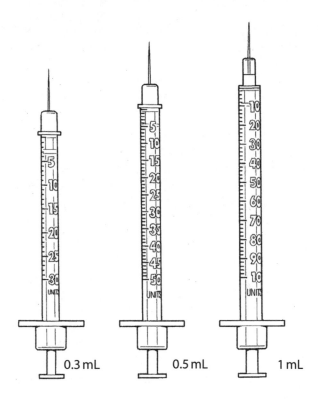

Figure 3.2 Insulin syringes: 0.3 mL, 0.5 mL and 1 mL

What length of needle should I use on my insulin pen?

There are several lengths of needle available today ranging from 5 mm to 12.7 mm. As a rule, they are used as follows:

- the 5 or 6 mm needle for children and thin to normal weight adults without a lifted skin fold (this means injecting straight into the skin without pinching it first);

- the 8 mm for normal weight adults with a lifted skin fold (loosely pinched);

- the 12 or 12.7 mm needle for overweight adults also with a lifted skin fold.

Ask your healthcare professional for the needle length and injection technique the most appropriate for you.

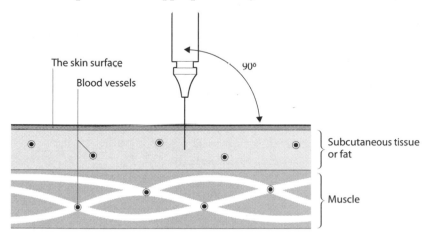

Figure 3.3 Skin layers

I am partially sighted. What pens or syringes are available for people like me, or for people who are blind? Are there any gadgets that would help me with my injections?

Most visually impaired people are advised to use an insulin pen rather than a syringe because you do not need to draw up insulin or check for air bubbles. The dialling mechanism usually has a distinctive clicking sound which reassures you that you have taken the correct dose. It is quite easy to use once the technique has been mastered, and offers a good choice of different types of insulin. This should be discussed with your physician or diabetes specialist nurse. There is a section *Insulin pens* earlier in this chapter.

Novo Nordisk produces a device called Innolet® that might well suit you. It is a disposable insulin pen with a large clock-like dial and a loud clicking sound with each unit dialled. It has raised spots at every 5 units marked. It also has a 'rocker' that allows you to rest the device on your skin before moving the needle forward to inject. It is easier to hold as it has a large grip.

Where should I keep my supplies of insulin?

Stores of insulin should ideally be kept in a refrigerator, but not in the freezer or freezing compartment. The ideal storage temperature is between 2° and 8°C. Below 0°C insulin is destroyed, and from 30°C upwards, insulin activity progressively decreases. If you do not have a fridge, then insulin may be stored for about a month at room temperature but keep it away from sources of direct heat such as radiators and strong sunlight. Many people prefer to keep their insulin bottle and/or their insulin pen that is in current use at room temperature as it may make the injection more comfortable (cold insulin increases the pain of the injection).

Should I wipe the top of the insulin bottle or insulin cartridge with spirit before use?

It is generally accepted that it is not necessary to clean the cartridge or insulin bottle top before use.

DIET AND INSULIN

My 16-year-old son has had diabetes since he was six. We have managed quite well but since he has been transferred to the diabetes clinic we have seen more of the dietitian. I am confused – she spends time urging us to eat more fibre-rich foods and cut down the fats. He's not overweight and has never had a problem with his bowels.

Your teenage son has now had his diabetes care transferred to the adult clinic. They will try to help your son become more involved in his diabetes care, as eventually he will have full responsibility for his own diabetes. This will include his choices of food and drink. The dietitian is leaning towards this independence by highlighting the guidelines for healthy eating (see the section *Diet*) which include encouraging carbohydrate foods which have a lower glycaemic index (see Table 3.3). These tend to be fibre-rich foods, such as oat-based cereals, fruit and vegetables and pulses. Reducing fat intake is also important as this can help protect against heart disease, and help to prevent unwanted weight gain, as your son matures to adulthood.

> *I understand that different forms of carbohydrate have different rates of digestion and that this affects the rise in blood glucose after a meal. I gather there is a 'glycaemic index' for each type of carbohydrate. What is this glycaemic index?*

The glycaemic index (GI) is a measure of how quickly foods that contain carbohydrate raise blood glucose levels. Each food is given a number relating to its effect on blood glucose. Foods with a high GI are quickly converted to glucose when eaten and cause a sharp rise in blood glucose levels. Foods with a low GI are converted to glucose much more slowly and produce a more gradual rise in blood glucose. The GI only tells us how quickly a food raises blood glucose when it is eaten on its own and as we usually eat a combination of foods this can change the overall GI of a meal. We do not recommend cutting out all foods with a high GI because your diet needs to be appealing as well as balanced. Low GI foods are generally more filling and can help control hunger as well as blood glucose levels, so they may help with weight loss. You need to be aware that the portion of carbohydrate is also important so eating large quantities of low GI foods can still affect your overall control. Some low GI foods, such as crisps and chocolate, are higher in fat and calories, so choices have to be made sensibly.

Knowing which foods have a high GI can be helpful for treating hypos as these will raise blood glucose more quickly. Table 3.3 gives

Table 3.3 Glycaemic index – a short table

Different tables may give slightly different results depending on the analysis.

Low GI foods (55 or less)	Medium GI foods (56–69)	High GI foods (70 or more)
All-Bran®, porridge made with water (42), Special K® (54)	muesli (56), Weetabix® (69), Shredded Wheat®	Bran flakes, Rice Krispies®, cornflakes, puffed wheat
multigrain breads, stoneground wholemeal bread (53)	wholemeal bread (69), pitta bread, rye bread	white bread, bagels, French bread, gluten-free bread
lentils, barley, kidney beans, butter beans, baked beans, chickpeas, peas, nuts*		broad beans
sweet potato, crisps (54)*	boiled potatoes	mashed potatoes, jacket potatoes, chips, parsnips
cherries, plums, apples, grapefruit, peaches, kiwi fruit, oranges, grapes, berries, bananas (55), mangoes (55)	sultanas, raisins, fruit tinned in syrup ripe bananas	watermelon, dates
wheat pasta, spaghetti, macaroni	basmati rice	white rice, rice pasta
milk, yoghurts, milk chocolate* (49)	ice-cream	jelly beans, jelly babies*

*although these foods have a low GI, it is due to their high fat content and so they are high in calories.
(numbers in brackets give GI of a certain food)

the GI of some popular foods. The website: www.glycaemicindex.com will give you more information on glycaemic index.

How long before eating should I have my insulin injection?

People who do not have diabetes start to produce insulin at the very beginning of a meal. If you are taking one of the fast-acting analogue insulins such as Humalog® or NovoRapid®, which mimic the action of natural insulin, it should be injected just before the meal. Some people prefer to inject immediately after the meal, when they know exactly how much they have eaten. There is evidence that the analogue insulins keep track of the rise in blood glucose better if given just before you eat.

If you take an insulin based on one of the older soluble insulins (e.g. Actrapid, Humulin S, Mixtard) or an animal insulin, you should aim to have your injection 20–30 minutes before your meal. If your blood glucose level is low you should delay your injection until you are ready to eat.

I am on two injections a day. Sometimes I find it inconvenient to take my evening injection. Can I skip it and have a meal containing no carbohydrate?

It would not be a good idea to skip your second (evening) injection, as this would leave you without insulin cover overnight. As the effect of your morning injection wears off, your blood glucose levels will rise even if you have eaten no carbohydrate. Insulin pens are easy to carry and should make it relatively easy to inject in most situations. If you need more flexibility in your insulin regimen then speak to your diabetes specialist nurse, who could explain alternative regimens for you to consider.

Do people taking insulin need to eat snacks in between meals?

Sometimes they do. When the pancreas functions normally, it produces insulin 'on demand' when you eat and 'switches off' when the food has been used up. Injected insulin does not 'switch off' in this way. As injected insulin has a peak effect at certain times of the day, it is important for you to cover its action by eating a certain amount of carbohydrates, or you will have a hypo. It is worth remembering that the carbohydrates will last longer if they have a lower glycaemic index (usually rich in fibre), as they are more slowly absorbed (see Table 3.3).

If you are taking a normal insulin before meals, you could try a very short-acting insulin analogue, such as NovoRapid® or

Humalog®. These are designed to provide insulin for the following meal but not to have an effect between meals, so you can avoid snacks. There are many ways in which you can adjust your insulin regimen to suit the life you lead, so talk with your doctor or diabetes specialist nurse about these.

I have been told that as I take insulin, I need to eat a bedtime snack. Is this true?

It depends on which insulin regimen you are on and what level your blood glucose is at bedtime. If you are taking mixed insulin twice a day, you may need a *small* bedtime snack, such as a piece of toast, fresh fruit, small sandwich, a small bowl of cereal or a yoghurt. It is not advisable to go to bed with a blood glucose level of less than 7 mmol/litre. If it is lower than this you run the risk of having a hypo during the night. If you are on a regimen of a long-acting insulin and three short-acting insulin injections (basal bolus) a bedtime snack should not be necessary. If you do need a bedtime snack your insulin may need adjusting.

Should I increase my insulin over Christmas to cope with the extra food I shall be eating?

Yes, you can take extra insulin to cover the extra carbohydrates that you eat on any special occasion, not just Christmas. At Christmas most people eat more and this is fine. Extra carbohydrate foods will need extra insulin and some trial and error may be required to achieve the correct increase in your dose. It would be safer to increase your insulin by a small amount (e.g. one to two units) at a time, unless you have experience of how much extra you require.

Is it all right for me to have a lie in on Sunday or must I get up and have my injection and breakfast at the normal time?

Your insulin treatment needs to fit your chosen lifestyle as much as possible and you should be able have a lie in on a Sunday if you wish! Some trial and error might be necessary and we would encourage you to monitor to see what works for you. If you are on twice-daily insulin and you delay your first injection by several hours, you may need to reduce this first dose, especially if you are having breakfast and lunch as one meal. If you are taking long-acting insulin first thing in the morning, it may be possible to change the timing of this insulin permanently to allow you the flexibility of lying in when you choose. If you only take short-acting insulin in the morning, it is much easier to omit this insulin and miss breakfast. You should make an appointment with your diabetes specialist nurse to discuss the options of changing your insulin regimen to suit your lifestyle.

I have two injections a day: morning and evening. I keep regular times for breakfast and evening tea but I would like to vary the time that I take lunch. What effect would this have on the control of my diabetes?

As you are taking two injections a day, it is most likely you are on a mixed insulin or a medium-acting insulin. Because insulins have a peak of activity, it is important that you cover this peak with food or you will increase your risk of a hypo. If you are having a later lunch you may have to include a mid-morning snack and be prepared to increase this to avoid a pre-lunch hypo. Trial and error and careful monitoring will give you the best guide to how much you can alter the timing of your lunch. If you feel you need more flexibility of mealtimes, multiple injections may be a better alternative for you. Your diabetes team can discuss options with you.

Sometimes I suffer from a poor appetite. Is it all right for me to reduce my insulin dose on such occasions?

The answer to this question depends on the number of insulin injections you take each day. If you use basal bolus insulin, it is easy to omit or reduce your mealtime insulin to match your food intake. You should never omit the long-acting dose. If you take insulin twice a day, and your appetite is reduced, you are at risk of a hypo if you miss a meal completely. It is never easy to deal with a variable or erratic meal pattern if you are on premixed insulin, but you could consider reducing the dose, using blood tests to help you decide how much insulin to take. If your appetite continues to be poor, or if you are losing weight unintentionally, you should see a dietitian for advice about food choices when your appetite is poor.

My daughter has had diabetes for four years and has had no problems with her diet. She takes part in most school sports but, since she has taken up running longer distances, she finds that she has a hypo about two hours after she has finished running. She has no problems during the run so what should she do to counteract this?

The effect of exercise on the body can last well after the exercise has stopped, as the muscles are restocking their energy stores with glycogen. Your daughter is obviously taking in enough food to last her during her run, but not enough to keep her going through this 'restocking' process. She would probably find it helpful to eat an extra carbohydrate snack, such as a fruit juice and a sandwich, after her run has finished. It might also be worth trying a small reduction in her morning dose of insulin on the days she is running. There is more about balancing insulin, food and exercise in the section *Sports* in Chapter 5.

My son has been putting on weight since being diagnosed as having diabetes three months ago. What are the reasons for this?

Most people lose weight before their diabetes is diagnosed and treated. In uncontrolled diabetes, body fat is broken down and many calories are lost as glucose in the urine (this is discussed in more detail in the section *Symptoms* in Chapter 1). As soon as the diabetes is brought under control, the body fat stops being broken down, the calories are no longer lost and the weight loss stops. Many people, like your son, begin to put weight back on again.

If your son starts to put on too much weight, he should discuss this with his diabetes specialist nurse and his dietitian. They will advise him about his diet and activity and about how ro reduce his food intake and insulin simultaneously.

There is a particular risk of weight gain when children stop growing. Children need larger amounts of food when they are actually growing taller, but once fully grown it is sensible to recommend ways of reducing their total calorie intake, for example by reducing fat intake. Girls usually stop growing a year or two after their first period and unless they start to change some of their eating habits at this stage they will run the risk of putting on weight – and it seems much easier to put on weight than to take it off.

I have been taking insulin for eight years and over this time I have put on a lot of weight. My doctor says that insulin does not make you fat, but if that is so, why have I put on so much weight?

Before starting insulin people often lose weight. This is because when diabetes is not controlled you lose lots of calories as glucose in the urine (see the section *Symptoms* in Chapter 1). When diabetes is controlled, the calories are no longer lost in the urine and the weight loss stops. There is then a tendency for people to put on weight or regain the weight they had lost. Insulin in the correct dose should not make you fat but if you are having too much insulin you have to eat more to prevent hypos. These extra calories will increase your weight. Also initially insulin can increase your appetite, as it lowers your blood glucose.

Trying to lose weight when you are on insulin is possible, but needs to be done slowly, as you cannot make drastic diet changes without upsetting your diabetes control. With careful reduction of both food and insulin, weight loss can be achieved but requires patience and perseverance (see the questions on Overweight, p. 29).

Since I went onto multiple injections to improve my control and fit in with my hectic work schedule I have put on quite a lot of weight. I am really pleased with my control and no longer miss insulin to avoid hypos but why do I keep on getting fatter?

Your change in insulin regimen is helping you control your diabetes and fits in better with your work. It is good that you are not missing your insulin and that there is a better match with your insulin and food intake. Since you are now able to use all the food you eat, any excess you do not need will be stored as fat.

To control your weight you need to balance the food you eat with the amount of energy you use up. Have a careful look at your diet. Perhaps you are choosing a sensible, healthy diet but your portions are too large.

If you are keen to reduce your weight, start by looking at the amounts of fat and alcohol in your diet, as these are both very concentrated sources of calories. Aim to cut back on any fatty foods, choosing low fat products instead of full fat, and having fruit or a diet yoghurt instead of crisps or biscuits as snacks. Choose lean meat, fish or poultry with the skin removed or Quorn. Include plenty of vegetables. You should aim for a weight loss of between 0.5–1 kg (1–2 lb) a week. If you are not making progress you may have to consider reducing your intake of starchy foods, along with blood glucose monitoring and reduction of your insulin to prevent hypos. Regular exercise will also help use up some of the excess calories. If your weight continues to be a problem, record all your meals and snacks for three or four days and then ask the dietitian to go over them with you to see where further changes can be made.

My 18-year-old daughter has diabetes and is trying to lose weight. She eats a low-carbohydrate diet and sticks to this rigidly. I cannot understand why she does not lose any weight.

Reducing a single food group, such as carbohydrate, in her diet will not necessarily lead to a loss of weight. Low carbohydrate diets are often much higher in fats and proteins so the total calories consumed are not necessarily reduced. A better and healthier approach would be to look carefully at what she eats and aim to reduce the higher calorie foods such as fatty foods and alcohol. Avoiding fried foods, using low fat dairy products, taking moderate amounts of protein as low fat meat, fish, chicken or meat substitutes such as tofu or Quorn, increasing fruit and vegetables, choosing carbohydrate foods with a lower glycaemic index, and including some regular activity would be the best long-term plan. Your daughter may benefit from help and support from a dietitian or diabetes specialist nurse.

I have heard that there is an anti-obesity pill that works by stopping fat absorption. Would it be suitable for me? I have diabetes and am very overweight.

The tablet you are probably referring to is called Xenical®, the brand name for orlistat. It blocks the digestion of fat and is the first anti-obesity pill not to rely on suppressing appetite. Orlistat manipulates the chemical digestion processes, blocking the action of lipases (enzymes that break up fat in the intestine), so that about 30% of fat in any meal goes undigested. However, there can be unpleasant side effects. The dietary fat that is not absorbed will be rapidly excreted, which can lead to stomach cramps, diarrhoea and 'oily spotting'. Orlistat is recommended for people with diabetes and if you manage to lose weight, it will help your diabetic control. The company has a very useful helpline which provides a whole package of advice about lifestyle. People who make use of the helpline are much more likely to succeed with orlistat.

HYPOS

I have had diabetes for 15 years and went straight onto insulin. I have always had plenty of warning when my sugars go low, but recently I had a bad hypo without any warning. My wife couldn't get me out of it and had to call the paramedics. This has rocked my confidence and I am afraid to aim at tight control of my blood sugars. Can you help?

There has been a lot of research into this problem of loss of warning of hypos – or 'hypo unawareness' as it is called. The first time a person becomes hypo, the body regards this as a very major threat since the brain cannot work properly without a normal supply of glucose. It reacts as it would to any serious threat by pouring out adrenaline – the 'fight and flight' hormone – which leads to many of the warning signs of a hypo, namely palpitations, sweating and panicky feelings (see Table 3.4). However, if people have repeated hypos, the body learns that the low blood glucose is not as dangerous as it first feared and the adrenaline response becomes blunted. Thus the most common cause of hypo unawareness is repeatedly running your blood glucose below normal. Several researchers have confirmed that hypo unawareness results from loss of the adrenaline response. The good news is that the warning signs will recover if you strictly keep your blood glucose above 4 mmol/L for at least four weeks. This means that you must take care to avoid low blood glucose in the night, when you may not realise that it is happening.

Table 3.4 Symptoms of a 'hypo'

Cause	Symptom
Adrenaline response	Sweating
	Pounding heart
	Shaking/trembling
	Hunger
	Anxiousness
	Tingling
Brain's lack of glucose	Confusion/difficulty in thinking
	Drowsiness/weakness
	Odd ('stroppy') behaviour
	Speech difficulty
Non-specific	Nausea
	Headache
	Tiredness

Since my partner has been started on insulin she has had funny turns. What is the cause of this?

Your partner's funny turns are likely to be due to a low blood glucose level. The medical term is hypoglycaemia; most people call it 'hypo' for short. When the blood glucose falls below a certain level (usually 3 mmol/litre), the brain is affected. Highly dependent on glucose, the brain stops working properly and begins to produce symptoms such as weakness of the legs, double or blurred vision, confusion, headache and, in severe cases, loss of consciousness and convulsions. Hypoglycaemia will also trigger the production of adrenaline, a hormone responsible for causing sweating, rapid heartbeat and feelings of panic and anxiety. Children often describe a 'dizzy feeling' or just 'tiredness' when they are hypoglycaemic. Most people find it hard to describe how they feel when hypo but the proof is that the blood glucose is low. If there is any doubt about the accuracy of your meter readings and you are feeling odd, it is always safer to take glucose or sugar. Symptoms of hypoglycaemia are shown in Table 3.4.

What is the best thing to take when I have a hypo?

This very much depends at which stage you recognise the hypo is developing. In the early stages the best treatment would be to have a meal or snack if one is due, or if there is some time before your next meal, an extra snack such as fruit, a sandwich or biscuits.

If your hypo is fairly well advanced, you need to take some very rapidly-absorbed carbohydrates. This is best taken as sugar, sweets or fruit juice or, for even greater speed, a sugary drink such as ordinary (not 'diet') cola, lemonade or Lucozade®. Good things to carry in your pocket are also glucose tablets such as Dextro-Energy as they are absorbed very quickly (three tablets of Dextro-Energy contain 10 g of glucose). They are also less likely to be eaten when you are not hypo than ordinary sweets!

You should eat some bread, biscuits or a small sandwich after the sugar or sugary drink.

I am taking soluble and isophane insulin twice a day and am getting hypos two to three hours after my evening meal. As I live alone this has been worrying me. What can I do?

Anyone who is having frequent hypos at a particular time of day can easily put this right by adjusting their insulin dose. In this case, you are having hypos at the time when your evening dose of soluble insulin is working. You should reduce the amount of soluble insulin you take in the evening until you have stopped having hypos at that time. On the other hand, hypos before your evening meal could be corrected by reducing your morning dose of intermediate-acting (isophane) insulin.

My teenage daughter has diabetes and sometimes turns very nasty and short-tempered. Is this due to the insulin?

Possibly – but of course there may be other reasons for bad moods. The only way to find out is to try to persuade her to have a blood glucose measurement during her bad moods. If it is low (4 mmol/L or less) then she is experiencing a hypo and some glucose should restore her good nature. Because the brain is affected by a low blood glucose level, irrational behaviour is common during a hypo. Your daughter may forcibly deny that she is hypo and resist taking the glucose her body needs. If you are firm and do not panic you will be able to talk her into taking the glucose (Lucozade®, lemonade or cola can be useful here) and she will soon be back to normal.

Children and adults can also become irritable if their blood glucose is very high.

My 8-year-old son often complains of feeling tired after recovering from a hypo. Is this usual and what is the best way to overcome it?

It is unusual to feel tired for more than 30 minutes after a hypo but, if your son does so, you should first check his blood glucose. If this is more than 4 mmol/L you will just have to let him rest until he is back to normal. It is not uncommon for hypos to trigger headaches and migraine attacks, which may be the problem here.

My teenage son refuses to take extra carbohydrate when he is hypo and insists that we let him sleep it off. Is this all right?

Hypos should always be corrected as quickly as possible. Your son is right in thinking that the insulin will eventually wear off and that his blood glucose will return to normal. However, if his blood glucose falls to very low levels, it could cause problems and he may even become unconscious. His refusal to take sugar is part of the confusion that occurs during a hypo and, if he can be persuaded to take glucose, he will get better more quickly.

I have been taking insulin for 38 years and my hypos have always been mild. Recently I suffered two blackouts lasting a minute, which I presume were hypos. Why has this started?

Blackouts tend to occur in children who have not yet learned to recognise the warning signs of a hypo but, on rare occasions, anyone on insulin can be caught unawares and have a sudden hypo, which makes them black out.

Sometimes as people get older the adrenaline warnings of a hypo fail to operate. This failure may be due to the natural ageing process or to damage (caused by diabetes) of the involuntary nerve supply which transmits the warning signs. Recent studies have suggested that keeping blood glucose levels above 4 mmol/L can help to restore lost hypo warnings. 'Make four the floor' is the advice given.

A number of people have also reported that after changing to human insulin they have less warning of hypos. So far there is no explanation for this. We have discussed human insulin in the section *Types of insulin* at the beginning of this chapter.

I have recently lost my warning signs for hypos. Is it likely that they will return?

Very tight diabetic control is known to reduce hypoglycaemic awareness. A study carried out with the help of people who had lost their warning symptoms showed that when the participants kept their blood glucose above 4 mmol/L continuously for three months, avoiding hypos altogether, they experienced partial or complete restoration of warning symptoms. Do you think that your diabetes could be too tightly controlled? If so, it may be worth discussing this with your diabetes team and reducing your dose of insulin.

My father has had diabetes for 20 years. Recently he had what his doctor calls epileptic fits. Would you tell me how to help him and if there is a cure?

A bad hypo may bring on a fit and it is important to check your father's blood glucose during an attack. If the glucose level is low, reducing his insulin should stop the fits. If the fits are not due to a low blood glucose level, it should be possible to control them by making sure he takes his epilepsy tablets regularly – ask his doctor for more details about these.

Can insulin reactions eventually cause permanent brain damage?

Many people ask about this as it is a great source of anxiety. The brain recovers quickly from a hypo and there is unlikely to be permanent damage, even after a severe attack with convulsions. Very prolonged hypoglycaemia can occur in someone with a tumour that produces insulin, and if a person is unconscious for days on end then the brain will not recover completely. This is not likely to occur in people with diabetes, in whom the insulin wears off after a few hours. However, there is some evidence that people who have very frequent hypos over many years may be at greater risk of dementia in later life.

If someone on insulin becomes very depressed, would they be able to commit suicide by taking an overdose of insulin?

Without dealing with the moral aspect of this question, we would strongly advise anyone against trying to commit suicide using insulin. It may sometimes lead to a painless death by hypoglycaemia but we know several cases where the person in question has lowered their blood glucose to dangerous levels for enough time to cause permanent brain damage but not to the level where it will lead to death. Most long-term brain injury units have one or two patients who are there because of a failed attempt to end their lives using insulin and this is a very sad situation for both the person concerned and for those close to them.

> *I have heard that there is an opposite to insulin called glucagon. Is this something like glucose and can it be used to bring someone round from a hypo?*

Glucagon is a hormone which, like insulin, is produced by the pancreas. It causes glucose to be released into the bloodstream from stores of starch in the liver. Glucagon can also be injected to bring someone round from a hypo if they are unconscious or too restless to swallow glucose. Glucagon cannot be stored in solution like insulin. It comes in a kit containing a vial with glucagon powder plus a syringe and sterile fluid for dissolving the powder. The process of dissolving the glucagon and drawing it into the syringe may be difficult, especially if you are feeling panicky. It is worth asking the diabetes specialist nurse to show you and your likely helper how to draw up glucagon.

Glucagon only has a short-lasting effect and it is therefore important to follow it up with some sugar by mouth to prevent a relapse of coma. When children have a glucagon injection their blood glucose level may rise sharply and make them feel sick, so they won't want more sugar. It is best to do a blood test to help decide whether more glucose is really needed immediately. More sustaining carbohydrates (such as bread or biscuits) should be given as soon as they feel well enough to eat, as the blood glucose level can fall again later.

> *When I gave my girlfriend a glucagon injection recently, she vomited. Is this normal?*

Some people do vomit when regaining consciousness after a glucagon injection, particularly children. If only half the content of the vial is given (0.5 mg), it will usually be enough to correct the hypo, but less likely to cause sickness.

What can I do if my son has a bad hypo and is too drowsy to take any glucose by mouth?

You should try giving him Glucogel (previously known as Hypostop). This is a gel loaded with glucose, which comes in a container with a nozzle. It can be squirted onto the gums of someone who is severely hypo and often leads to recovery within a few minutes. Glucogel is available on prescription from your GP, or can be obtained from Bio-Diagnostics Ltd (the address is in Appendix 2). If Glucogel fails, you should try injecting your son with glucagon – there are some questions about glucagon above.

My daughter aged 21 takes insulin for her diabetes and is moving down to London where she hopes to rent a flat on her own. In view of the risk of hypoglycaemic attacks, would you advise against this?

By the age of 21 your daughter will be ready to be independent and live in a flat by herself. All parents worry when their children leave home, and diabetes adds to their anxiety, but sooner or later young people have to lead separate lives. We know that night hypos are common and that either people wake up and sort themselves out or else their blood glucose returns to normal as the insulin wears off and they wake up next morning unaware of any problem. However, there have been a handful of cases when people on insulin are found dead in bed, and it is possible that some of these are due to hypoglycaemia. This must be a cause of concern but considering the hundreds of thousands of people on insulin, the risk of this tragedy is like that of being struck by lightning.

Your daughter should be aware of the risk of hypo when driving or swimming and be encouraged to tell her close friends and companions about diabetes. They should be told that, if ever she behaves oddly, she must be given some form of sugar, even if she protests. This simple precaution can avoid a lot of worry to friends who may find people hypo and have no idea how to help.

4 | Monitoring and control

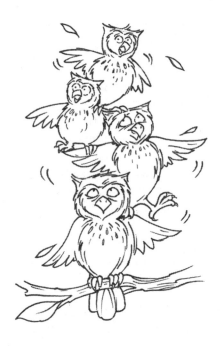

Successful diabetes control means achieving good blood glucose levels without hypos. The fact that you feel well does not necessarily mean that your blood glucose is satisfactory. You only feel unwell if your sugar is either well above normal or too low. If it is low, you may be aware of hypo symptoms – if left untreated this may progress to unconsciousness (hypoglycaemic coma). At the other end of the spectrum, when the blood glucose is very high, you may be aware of increased thirst and passing urine excessively – left untreated, this may progress to nausea, vomiting, weakness, and eventual clouding of consciousness and coma (a condition called ketoacidosis). It has long been apparent that relying on how you feel is too imprecise, even though some people may be able to 'feel' subtle changes in their control. For this reason, many different tests have been developed to allow precise measurement of control and, as the years go by, these tests become more efficient and accurate.

The involvement of the person with diabetes in monitoring and control of their own condition has always been essential for successful treatment. With the development of blood glucose monitoring, this has become even more apparent: it allows you to measure precisely how effective you are at balancing the conflicting forces of diet, exercise and insulin, and to make adjustments in order to maintain this balance. In the early days after the discovery of insulin, urine tests were the only tests available and it required a small laboratory even to do these. Urine tests have always had the disadvantage that they are only an indirect indicator of what you really need to know, which is the level of glucose in the blood. Blood glucose monitoring first became available to people with diabetes in 1977 and is now widely accepted. As anyone who has monitored glucose levels in the blood will know, these vary considerably throughout the day as well as from day to day. For this reason, a single reading at a twice yearly visit to the local diabetes clinic is of limited value in assessing long-term success or failure with control.

The introduction of haemoglobin A_{1c} (glycosylated haemoglobin or HbA_{1c}) has provided a very reliable test for longer-term monitoring of average blood glucose levels (taking into account the peaks and troughs) over an interval of two to three months. Someone with diabetes should aim at a target HbA_{1c} of 6.5–7.5%, which indicates that the blood glucose has been contained within the near normal range. Provided there have been no troublesome hypoglycaemic attacks, this means that balance of diabetes has been excellent and no further changes are required. Achieving a normal HbA_{1c} level and maintaining it as near normal as possible is an important goal. Not everyone can achieve this, but it is undoubtedly the most effective way of eliminating the risk of long-term complications.

The importance of good blood glucose control in preventing complications has been proven for Type 1 diabetes in the Diabetes Control and Complications Trial (DCCT) in the USA. In this painstaking study over 1400 people with Type 1 diabetes were divided into two groups, depending on how closely they controlled their blood glucose, and then followed up for an average of seven years.

The group with good control, with an average HbA$_{1c}$ of 7.2% (see the section *Haemoglobin A$_{1c}$* later in this chapter for an explanation of this measurement) benefited from a 60% reduction in disease of the eyes, kidneys and nerves compared with the group with worse control. To achieve this degree of control, the people in this group had four daily injections or received insulin via a constant infusion pump. They also had considerable support from a team of diabetes specialists, including nurse educators, dietitians, psychologists and doctors. The group with tight control also had a greater risk of hypos (see section *Hypos* in Chapter 3).

WHY MONITOR?

I am an 18-year-old on insulin. When my glucose is high I do not feel any ill effects. Does it really matter what my sugar level is?

It is quite true that some people do not develop the typical thirst or dry mouth, frequency of passing water (urination), or tiredness, which usually occur if the blood glucose is high and diabetes out of control. If you lack these warning signs, control of your diabetes will be more difficult as there will be no direct motivation to keep your blood glucose normal. However, people who consistently run high blood glucose levels carry a greater risk of developing complications of diabetes. On the other hand if you manage to keep your glucose level near normal, you make the risk of complications much less and may even eliminate it. We know that it is difficult at 18 to be concerned about things that might only happen a long time ahead in your future, but good control really is worth it in the long run.

My 17-year-old daughter has had diabetes for six years. She is finding it very difficult to keep her diabetes under control at present and doesn't seem to care if her sugars run high most of the time. Do you think she is doing herself any real damage?

There is now strong evidence that good control of blood glucose reduces the risk of developing the complications of diabetes (which are dealt with in Chapter 9) and this was confirmed in September 1993 when the results of the Diabetes Control and Complications Trial (DCCT) were published (see the introduction to this chapter). This improvement in control was achieved at a cost, with a three-fold increase in the risk of hypos in the good control group. Some of these hypos required help from someone else to bring the person round.

Thus your daughter is faced with a difficult decision. If she carries on with poor control, she increases her chance of developing long-term problems from her diabetes. If, on the other hand, she decides to try to improve her blood glucose levels, she may have more hypos. It would be worth spending time with your daughter helping her to realise that although the recommended target for HbA_{1c} is 6.5–7.5%, any improvement is worthwhile. More recently we have learned that most people can improve control without their life being disrupted by hypos. Your daughter should be encouraged to take part in an education course such as DAFNE (see next question), which would help improve control and put her in touch with other people with Type 1 diabetes who are grappling with the same problem.

A friend from work who has had diabetes for years took a week off to do a diabetes course called DAFNE. Since coming back, he has been raving about it. Could you please let me know more about it?

Most people who take part in the DAFNE programme find it a useful and sometimes life-changing experience. The idea of intensive education was developed in Dusseldorf, Germany by Michael Berger and Ingrid Muhlhauser, two specialists in diabetes with an interest in patient education. They had been inspired by Jean Philippe Assal, a Swiss doctor with Type 1 diabetes who pioneered a new method of patient education. The German course was residential and people with Type 1 diabetes spent a week learning about diabetes. In 1998, a group of diabetes specialists from England went to observe the Dusseldorf course and were very impressed by the method of teaching and the enthusiasm of both the educators and the participants. With help from Michael and Ingrid they designed a British version, which they called DAFNE (Dose Adjustment For Normal Eating). They carried out a formal research project which was published in 2002. This showed that the 5-day course improved blood glucose control, quality of life and treatment satisfaction. There are now 37 DAFNE centres in the UK and Ireland with another 19 in training.

DAFNE allows more dietary freedom by teaching people to calculate how much insulin they need for the food they plan to eat. This means that foods such as cake or puddings, which are normally restricted, can be eaten whenever desired as long as enough insulin is taken to prevent the blood glucose from rising. With practice, people become very skilled at calculating the amount of insulin required and there is good evidence that the DAFNE method can improve control, reduce hypos and allow more flexible eating.

DAFNE is not the only course for people with Type 1 diabetes. There are a number of others in various parts of the country and you should ask your local diabetes centre what they can offer. Diabetes UK has recommended ways of assessing education courses and you can access this information from their website.

I have heard good reports of the DAFNE course and would like to take part in it. However, I don't think my local hospital does the course. What can I do about this?

It is unfortunate that however much the government tries to abolish 'postcode prescribing' there are still great variations in resources in different parts of the country. Even if a DAFNE centre is established in a hospital, there may still be problems with funding the courses. There are now 37 DAFNE centres in England, Scotland, Wales and Ireland with another 19 in training. However, many diabetes centres have developed their own education package for people with Type 1 diabetes. A phone call to the hospital diabetes centre will tell you if there is any such provision. If not, you could ask your GP to refer you to a DAFNE centre, but this would require funding to cover the costs of the programme. If you have access to the internet, the DAFNE website (www.dafne.uk.com) can provide full information about the project.

Whenever I go to the clinic I always feel guilty for not doing enough blood tests. I have had diabetes for ten years – since I was 25 years old. I sometimes feel like writing some make-believe tests into my testing book just to keep the doctors happy.

Writing make-believe tests in your book won't keep your doctors happy and, more importantly, won't stop you feeling guilty about not doing your blood tests. What might help is looking at some possible reasons why you are not doing the tests.

When you first went on insulin you were probably the centre of attention with support from your family, school friends or workmates. You probably had close contact with a diabetes specialist nurse to help you through this difficult time. During this period, measuring your blood glucose became a routine occurrence so that you could adjust your dose of insulin. After becoming more confident with your diabetes, you may have decided on a fixed insulin dose, which you only vary under unusual circumstances.

It can be depressing when the initial interest fades and you have to come to terms with the fact that the routine of diabetes will never go away. This is a time when people may stop doing regular blood tests. We have interviewed a number of people who have given up testing and these are the most common reasons they give.

- Testing is messy and bloody.
- I haven't got time/can't be bothered to test my blood.

- There is no need to test if you feel all right.

- Testing my blood brings it home to me that I have diabetes.

- It is inconvenient/embarrassing to test in public or at work.

- Insulin injections are essential, blood tests are not.

- A bad test makes me feel even more depressed about my diabetes.

- There is no point in testing my blood as I don't use the information.

These are the opinions of people living with diabetes and they must be respected. You might like to think about where you stand on this subject, and perhaps discuss it with someone on your next clinic visit. We believe that you will only achieve good control by doing regular blood tests since there is no other way of knowing exactly where you are with your diabetes.

In the past 12 months I have had to increase my insulin dosage several times, but have been unable to get a blood test result that was near normal. I have had diabetes for 25 years and until last year I have always been well controlled. What has gone wrong?

Here are a few reasons why your blood glucose levels may have crept up and why you need more insulin after many years of good control:

- less exercise, meaning that more insulin is needed for your food intake;

- an increase in the amount of food you eat;

- increased stress or emotional upsets;

- any illness that lingers on, leading to a need for more insulin;

- technical problems with injections such as the appearance of lumps from repeated doses of insulin into the same site;

- increase in weight and middle-age spread;

- treatment with certain drugs, especially steroids.

Apart from these identified reasons, some people do find that the dose of insulin that they need may vary by quite large amounts with no obvious explanation.

Can stress influence blood glucose readings?

Yes, but the response varies from one person to another. In some people stress tends to make the blood glucose rise whereas in other people it may increase the risk of hypoglycaemia.

BLOOD GLUCOSE MONITORING

My GP says blood tests are very expensive and wants me to cut down the number of tests. I take insulin with each meal and at bedtime to control my diabetes. How often should I be testing?

There is great pressure on GPs to reduce their spending on drugs and since blood glucose testing strips are very expensive, these are often selected as a target for cutting costs. Most strips cost around £28 for 50. Those doctors and pharmacists who want to restrict the number of test strips prescribed, often point to people with diabetes who test their blood glucose very regularly but do not make use of the results. In such people, blood testing has become a way of life, which provides reassurance but does not alter day-to-day insulin doses.

As someone who takes insulin with every meal, you probably want to make a decision about how much insulin to take, based on what you are about to eat and the level of your pre-meal blood glucose. You will therefore want to test at least four times a day. Many people who take insulin twice a day do not adjust their insulin on a daily basis so frequent blood testing becomes less important. Our local Primary Care Trust, which is responsible for advising GPs about economical prescribing, has agreed blood glucose monitoring guidelines which appear in Figure 4.1. The number of tests recommended depends on the type and frequency of insulin injections and may range from once to six times a day. It is important to remember that the DVLA regulations state that people taking insulin *must* test before they drive.

Figure 4.1

BLOOD GLUCOSE SELF-MONITORING GUIDELINES *These guidelines were developed by Coventry PCT*		
Education and lifestyle interventions	• Advice on diet, exercise and smoking are key interventions at diagnosis and beyond • If necessary, patients should receive education relevant to **appropriate** testing, **understanding when** to test and **what** to do with the result	ALL PATIENTS WHO ARE SELF-MONITORING SHOULD BE ENCOURAGED TO USE THE MINIMUM NUMBER OF TESTS REQUIRED TO KEEP CONTROL
Newly diagnosed Type 2 patient + diet control only Recommended regime: A	• Self-monitoring may be required at diagnosis or as necessary depending on overall diabetic control and management plan • Self-monitoring may **not be necessary** if control is acceptable (e.g. HbA$_{1c}$ to target) • Healthcare professional should advise patient when self-monitoring becomes necessary	Urine testing may be appropriate for some patients in this group provided HbA$_{1c}$ targets are achieved Typical weekly strip usage 0–6

Type 2 patient, prescribed oral therapy Recommended regimes: A, B, C	• Re-assess patient need and educate prior to initiation of single oral therapy or combined treatment • If self-monitoring is necessary, the healthcare professional should tailor monitoring regime to individual patient need, depending on diabetic control • Special focus on testing to prevent hypoglycaemia, especially in sulphonylurea therapy	If starting self-monitoring at this stage teach patient before initiating new therapy	Typical weekly strip usage 0–6
Type 2 patient, prescribed insulin Recommended regimes: B, D, E	• Self-monitoring is recommended in all cases with daily testing on initiation of insulin • Once a patient is stable, frequency of profiles can be reduced to 1–2 days a week or daily at varying times (week profile)	Stable patients are those whose blood glucose varies little from day to day and who are not having intensive changes of treatment	Typical weekly strip usage 4–28
Type 1 patients Recommended regimes E, F	• Self-monitoring is strongly recommended in all cases • Self-monitoring should be used to adjust insulin dose before meals where this is appropriate (e.g. basal bolus regime, pump therapy) • Self-monitoring in Type 1 diabetes may only be required on 1–2 days per week in stable patients and depending on patient's daily routine		Typical weekly strip usage 8–28

Figure 4.1 (*continued*)

Examples of typical self-monitoring regimes

Regime A	One or two tests a week
Regime B	Once daily at various times (week profile)
Regime C	Two tests daily
Regime D	Four tests at different times on one day (day profile)
Regime E	Day profile twice a week
Regime F	Test before meals and at bedtime each day

- Urine testing is appropriate in those:
    where blood glucose monitoring is not possible
    or the patient has a preference not to blood test
- HbA$_{1c}$ target = below 7.5%
- Increase testing frequency during:
    pregnancy
    times of illness
    changes in therapy
    changes in routine
    times of poor control
    when at risk of hypoglycaemia
    also to rule out hypoglycaemia, especially when driving.

Blood glucose monitoring targets

Fasting	4–6 mmol/L	Bedtime	5–10 mmol/L
Pre-prandial	4–6 mmol/L	Post-prandial	<10 mmol/L

- Self-monitoring does not replace regular HbA$_{1c}$ testing , which remains the gold standard test, and should only be used in conjunction with appropriate therapy as part of integrated care.

What is the normal range of blood glucose in a person who does not have diabetes?

Before meals the range is from 3.5 to 5.5 mmol/litre. After meals it may rise as high as 10 mmol/L depending on the carbohydrate content of the meal. However long a person without diabetes goes without food, the blood glucose concentration never drops below 3 mmol/L, and however much they eat, it never goes above 10 mmol/L.

My blood glucose monitor is calculated in millimoles. What's a millimole?

In the 1960s, international agreement led scientists in most parts of the world to adopt a standard system of metric measurements. The units are called SI units, an abbreviation of their full name – the 'Système International d'Unites'. There are several units, many of which you probably use without thinking about them, such as the metre. The unit for an amount of a substance is called a mole; the prefix 'milli-' means one-thousandth, so a millimole is one-thousandth of a mole. Blood glucose is measured in millimoles of glucose per litre of blood, and this is abbreviated to mmol/L.

Before SI units were introduced, blood glucose was measured in milligrams per 100 millilitres of blood (abbreviated to mg% or to mg per dL) and this measurement is still used in the USA. Table 4.1 shows how one set of units relates to the other.

Should I keep my blood glucose monitoring sticks in the fridge with my insulin?

No. It is important to keep them dry as any moisture will affect their activity. The bottle of sticks should be kept in a cool, dry place, and not be exposed to extremely high temperatures. You must put the lid back on the container immediately after removing a strip (unless the strips are individually foil-wrapped). Many of the strips

Table 4.1 Blood glucose measurements

1 mmol/L = 18 mg%	2 mmol/L = 36 mg%
3 mmol/L = 54 mg%	4 mmol/L = 72 mg%
5 mmol/L = 90 mg%	6 mmol/L = 108 mg%
7 mmol/L = 126 mg%	8 mmol/L = 144 mg%
9 mmol/L = 162 mg%	10 mmol/L = 180 mg%
1 mmol/L = 216 mg%	15 mmol/L = 270 mg%
20 mmol/L = 360 mg%	22 mmol/L = 396 mg%
25 mmol/L = 450 mg%	30 mmol/L = 540 mg%

contain enzymes, which are biological substances that do not last forever, and the sticks should never be used beyond their expiry date. If you have any reason to suspect the result of a blood test, it is best to repeat the test using a new bottle of strips.

> *I feel hypo when my blood glucose is normal and only well when it is high. I feel very ill when my doctor tries to keep my blood glucose normal. Am I hooked on a high blood glucose?*

When you have had poor control for several years, the brain and other tissues in the body can adjust to a high concentration of glucose in the blood. As a result you may feel hypo at a time when your blood glucose is normal or even high. The long-term outlook for people in your situation is not good unless you can re-educate yourself to tolerate normal blood glucose levels without feeling unwell. This is possible but requires determination and an understanding of the long-term dangers of a high blood glucose.

Your problem can be overcome by regular measurement and a gradual lowering of your blood glucose so that your body has the chance to adjust to the lower levels. You must believe that, however unwell you feel, no harm will be done if your blood glucose remains above 4 mmol/litre. It may take up to six months for this re-education process to take effect, but it will be worth it.

Is there a way of knowing how much extra short-acting insulin to give depending on my blood glucose level so I can maintain a better blood glucose?

The DAFNE method (see p. 91) and other similar educational systems provide clear answers to your question. During the DAFNE course participants learn:

- How they react to the insulin they take;
- What carbohydrates are and how to estimate the carbohydrate content of different foods;
- How to calculate the amount of insulin they require to cover the carbohydrate in the food they are about to eat.

DAFNE also helps people to work out how much background insulin is required to control their blood sugar when they are in the basal condition, before eating food. If you are having the correct dose of background insulin and your blood glucose is unexpectedly high before a meal, DAFNE recommends that you take a 'corrective' added to your pre-meal insulin. This is normally calculated using the formula:

1 unit of short-acting insulin reduces your blood glucose by 3 mmol/L

Thus if your glucose is 12–14 and you feel it should be closer to 6, you should add 2 units of insulin as a corrective to the dose of mealtime insulin.

Are there any general guidelines for insulin adjustment?

If you have Type 1 diabetes, we would recommend that you try to enrol in a course designed to help people learn the principles of living with insulin. The first of these courses was DAFNE (see p. 91) but many diabetes centres run either DAFNE or similar courses.

> *I find that my control is only good for one week a month and that is the week before my period. Why is this and what should I do about it?*

In some women the dose of insulin required to control diabetes varies in relation to the menstrual cycle. Your question implies that you become more sensitive to insulin in the week before you menstruate and you probably require more insulin at the other times in your cycle. There is no reason why you should not try to work out a pattern where you reduce your insulin dose in the week before your period and increase it at other times.

The variation is due to different hormones coming from the ovaries during the menstrual cycle. Some of these hormones have an anti-insulin effect. The same sort of effects may occur when a woman is taking oral contraceptive tablets (the Pill) or is pregnant. You should try to make adjustments in the insulin dose in order to compensate for these hormonal changes and to keep the balance of the blood glucose where it should be. Your diabetes clinic doctor or diabetes specialist nurse is the best person to turn to for exact advice on how to make these adjustments.

> *I have been using Mixtard for years. I take 36 units before breakfast and 24 units before my evening meal. My blood tests are normally pretty good except for bedtime when they are often as high as 15 mmol/L. My doctor says my control is poor and wants me have more injections. What is your view on this?*

Twice daily injections of insulin are usually a compromise, especially in Type 1 diabetes, when there are no reserves of insulin. It sounds as if your evening dose does not supply enough short-acting insulin to cope with your evening meal, though the long-acting component of Mixtard is able to provide enough overnight background insulin. A fairly simple solution would be to 'split the evening dose'. You would have to take a dose of short-acting insulin before your evening meal and some background insulin at bedtime. The doses would have to be adjusted depending on the results of blood tests. This new arrangement would have the added advantage that you could vary the pre-meal dose of insulin depending on how much you wanted to eat.

Where is the best place to obtain blood for measuring blood glucose levels?

It is usually easiest to obtain blood from the fingertips. You can use either the pulp, which is the fleshy part of the fingertip, or the sides. The sides of the fingertips are less sensitive than the pulp. Some people use the area just below the nailbed. It may be necessary for people such as guitarists, pianists or typists to avoid the finger pulp.

Parents may find that it is easiest to obtain blood from the earlobes of their child with diabetes. There are a couple of meters that allow blood to be taken from the arm. (See the question on arm testing later in this chapter.)

Which is the best finger-pricking device?

All blood lancets (finger prickers) are very similar and there is little to choose between them. The lancets may be used either on their own or in conjunction with an automatic device. They are obtainable on prescription from your GP. Alternatively they can be bought from a chemist, or ordered by post from companies such as Owen Mumford (Medical Shop); see Appendix 2 for addresses.

The automatic devices work on the principle of hiding the lancet from view while piercing the skin very quickly and at a controlled depth. The meter you are using will have had an accompanying finger pricking device. They are not available on prescription, but can be obtained from the manufacturer of your meter (see Table 4.2) or by post from companies such as Owen Mumford (Medical Shop).

MORECAMBE BAY HOSPITALS NHS TRUST

Table 4.2 Blood glucose meters

Company	Meter name	Test strip name	Size of sample (in microlitres)	Range of results (in mmoles)	Test time (in seconds)
Abbott Diabetes care (helpline 0500 467 466)	Medisense Optium Xceed	Medisense Optium Plus Electrodes (also Medisense B ketone electrodes to measure blood ketone levels)	0.6	1.1–27.8	5
	Freestyle Freedom	Freestyle	0.3	1.1–27.8	5
	Freestyle Mini	Freestyle	0.3	1.1–27.8	7
ADL Healthcare Diagnostics (helpline 0800 08 588 08) truetrack@adlhealthcare.co.uk	TrueTrack SmartSystem	TrueTrack SmartSystem	1.0	1.3–33.3	10
Bayer HealthCare (helpline 0845 600 6030) www.ascensia.co.uk	Ascensia Contour	Ascensia Microfill Test Strips (10 test disc)	0.6	0.6–33.3	15
	Ascensia Breeze	Ascensia Autodisc (10 test disc)	2–3	0.6–33.3	30
CDx Ltd (helpline 0191 564 2036) www.cdx.uk.com	SensoCard Plus (Talking Meter)	SensoCard	0.5	1.1–33.3	5
LifeScan (helpline 0800 121 200) www.lifescan.co.uk	One Touch Ultra	One Touch Ultra Test Strips	1	1.1–33.3	5
	One Touch Ultra Smart	One Touch Ultra Test Strips	1	1.1–33.3	5

Company	Meter name	Test strip name	Size of sample (in microlitres)	Range of results (in mmoles)	Test time (in seconds)
Menarini	GlucoMen® Visio	GlucoMen® Visio Sensors	0.8	1.1–33.3	10
(helpline 0800 243 667)	GlucoMen® PC	GlucoMen® sensors	2.0	1.3–33.3	30
visio@menarinidiag.co.uk	GlucoMen® Glyco	GlucoMen® sensors	2.0	1.3–33.3	30
Roche Diagnostics	Accu-chek® Aviva	Accu-chek® Aviva	0.6	0.6–33.3	5
(helpline 0800 701 000)	Accu-chek® Active	Accu-chek® Active Strips	2	0.55–33.3	5
www.accu-chek.co.uk	Compact Plus	Compact Plus	1.5	0.55–33.3	5
	Accu-chek® Advantage	Advantage Plus	4	0.55–33.3	25

Should I clean my fingers with spirit or antiseptic before pricking them?

We do not recommend that you use spirit for cleaning your fingers. Spirit or antiseptic could interfere with the test strip and cause soreness if you have recently pricked the same finger. We suggest that you wash your hands with soap and warm water, or only water, and dry them thoroughly before pricking your finger. The main reason for having a clean finger is to remove any contamination, such as food, that may cause a false blood glucose result.

Will constant finger pricking make my fingers sore?

You may find that your fingers feel sore for the first week or two after starting blood glucose monitoring but this seems to settle down. We have seen many people who have been measuring their blood glucose levels regularly three or four times a day for more than 15 years and who have no problems with sore fingers. The more up-to-date meters use very small amounts of blood and so you don't need to prick your finger too brutally! Don't always use the same finger – try to use different fingers in turn.

Will my fingers take a long time to heal after finger pricking and am I more likely to pick up an infection there?

Your fingertips should heal as quickly as those of someone without diabetes, but make sure that you are using suitable blood lancets. We have seen only one infected finger among many hundreds of thousands of finger pricks. As long as your hands are clean when you take your blood sample, you should not have any problems.

There are a bewildering number of strips and meters on the market. Which are the best to use?

A few years ago most people were using strips without a meter. This required performing a complicated procedure in order to obtain an accurate blood glucose result. Now in the UK you can only use a strip with a meter. The meters are very similar in terms of reliability and performance. There are small differences, for example the amount of blood required to perform a test or the time it takes for the meter to produce the results (see Table 4.2). Nearly all the meters can be downloaded onto a PC and software is usually available free from the manufacturers.

Blood testing is not just about doing the test but making sense of the results. Your healthcare professional will show you how to use your meter, and you will need further time to discuss your results and what you might need to change in order to achieve the levels you want.

Blood glucose testing strips are available on prescription from your GP. The meters are quite inexpensive and may be available free from your diabetes nurse.

I have recently started testing my blood sugar levels but my results do not compare well with the clinic results. What is the reason for this?

It is not clear if your blood sugar results are being compared with blood glucose tests at the hospital or with another test known as the HbA_{1c}, glycosylated haemoglobin or long-term test. The HbA_{1c} is usually measured only once or twice a year. The test measures the amount of glucose that has attached itself to the red blood cells, throughout their 2–3 month life span (see section *Haemoglobin A_{1c}* later in this chapter). Research tells us that to avoid complications of diabetes the HbA_{1c} should be under 7.5% (see introduction to this chapter). The HbA_{1c} is often described as an average of blood glucose levels but strictly speaking it is not an average. For example, if your

HbA$_{1c}$ is 12% your blood glucose levels are likely to be averaging around 19 mmol/L. When you perform a blood glucose test at home you are measuring the result as it is at that minute in time. Two hours later it could be much lower or much higher. The HbA$_{1c}$ is not measuring the highs and lows but what has accumulated in the previous two to three months.

In summary, it is possible that your home blood glucose tests are being compared with the HbA$_{1c}$ which is a different kind of test. Alternatively, the blood is being tested at a different time or on a different blood testing machine, which can cause a variation in results.

Are the blood glucose meters accurate enough for daily use?

Most results obtained when you are using a meter will be slightly different from the clinic laboratory results or even from different makes of meters because different technological methods are used. These slight differences do not matter and the strips and meters are quite accurate enough for home use provided your technique is correct. If you are concerned that your results may not be accurate you can check the meter yourself by using the quality control solution provided with the meter. Phone the meter company helpline (see Table 4.2) for advice or contact your diabetes specialist nurse who can check both your meter and your technique.

I have heard that there is a watch you can wear that measures the blood sugar automatically. Is this right?

You are thinking about the GlucoWatch®, developed by a Californian company called Cygnus Inc. Unfortunately there were many technological problems and so the GlucoWatch is currently unavailable in the UK. This device is worn like a wristwatch and measures blood glucose from interstitial fluid every 10–20 minutes depending on the model. The watch had to be fitted with a sensor which only lasted for 12 hours and was expensive to buy.

I have heard that it is now possible to obtain a meter which can measure the blood glucose constantly without the need for repeated fingerpricks. How do I get hold of one?

Meters which provide a continuous read-out of blood glucose levels are available for research purposes and for short-term use. The eventual aim is to connect these meters to an insulin pump allowing the dose of insulin to be controlled by the level of blood glucose – a true 'artificial pancreas'. The technology is promising but not fully developed.

At present the Minimed Medtronic can record the blood glucose continuously for three days and many diabetes centres will own such a meter. They can be loaned to people who are having problems with their diabetes control and are used to identify patterns of either high or low blood glucose. They do not produce an immediate reading but can be downloaded to a computer to print out a three-day blood glucose curve. Unfortunately the three-day probes are expensive and are not yet practical for long term use.

I have trouble obtaining enough blood to perform a blood sugar test. Is there anything that I can do to make this easier?

The good news is that many of the new meters need only tiny amounts of blood in order to perform a test (see Table 4.2). However, if you are having trouble obtaining enough blood then try warming your hands by washing them in warm water before you start, and drying them thoroughly before pricking your finger. When squeezing the blood out of your finger, try 'milking' the blood out gently, allowing the finger to recover between each squeeze. Do not squeeze so hard that you blanch the finger white.

I am about to buy a meter that allows blood to be taken from the arm. Are there any problems with arm testing?

At the time of writing there are three meters that allow blood for testing to be taken from the arm. They are the OneTouch® Ultra from LifeScan and the FreeStyle® Freedom and Freestyle Mini from Abbott. The OneTouch Ultra and FreeStyle use strips that allow a tiny blood sample to be taken, which makes arm testing feasible. Under certain conditions, samples taken from the arm may differ significantly from fingertip samples, such as when blood glucose is changing rapidly:

- following a meal;
- after an insulin dose;
- when taking physical exercise.

Arm samples should only be used for testing *prior to*, or *more than two hours after* meals, an insulin dose or physical exercise. Fingertip testing should be used whenever there is a concern about hypoglycaemia (such as before you drive a car), as arm testing may not detect hypoglycaemia. Obtaining sufficient blood from the arm is not always easy but for some it is a welcome alternative to fingertip pricking. Your health professional should be consulted before you begin arm testing.

I have heard that there is a way of obtaining blood from a finger using a laser. Is this true?

The Lasette is a single shot laser that makes a small hole in the finger to obtain a drop of blood, but it is not a blood glucose monitoring device. The use of laser light, as opposed to a steel lancet, reduces tissue damage, and many users of the device report feeling less pain than when using a traditional lancet. It weighs just less than 260 g (9 oz). However, it is very expensive. It is slightly smaller than a videocassette. The Lasette is manufactured by Cell Robotics, and can be obtained from Nutech International, whose address is in Appendix 2.

I would like to measure my own blood glucose levels, but as I am blind I do not know if this is possible. Can it be done?

A fter a long spell when no speaking meters were available there is now the new SensoCard® Plus Meter which will speak instructions and also speak the result (see Table 4.2). The meter has recently come down in price. Strips are available on prescription and your pharmacist would need to contact the company, CDx Ltd, directly (address in Appendix 2). This company also supplies control solution to check that the meter is working properly, and software to download results from a computer.

URINE

How do you know if you have ketones in your urine? What are they and are they dangerous?

K etones are breakdown products of the fat stores in the body. They are present in small amounts even in people without diabetes, particularly when they are dieting or fasting and therefore relying on their body fat stores for energy. In people with diabetes small amounts of ketones in the urine are commonly found. They become dangerous only when they are present in large amounts. This is usually accompanied by thirst, passing large amounts of urine, and nausea. If ketones are present in the urine together with continuous 2% glucose, or blood glucose levels higher than 13 mmol/L, this could be a dangerous condition that precedes the development of ketoacidosis. *Under these circumstances you should seek urgent medical advice.*

You can test your urine for ketones with strips such as Ketur Test® or Keto Diabur®; the latter tests for glucose as well and both are made by Roche; or Ketostix® or KetoDiastix® (made by Bayer Diagnostics) – they are all available on prescription from your GP. MediSense produce an Optium® meter that tests for blood glucose and blood ketones but, although the glucose testing strips are available on prescription, the blood ketone strips are not.

What does it mean if I have a lot of ketones but no glucose on urine testing?

Testing for ketones in the urine can be rather confusing and, unless there are special reasons for doing it, we do not recommend it for routine use. Some people seem to develop ketones in the urine very readily, especially children, pregnant women and those who are dieting strictly to lose weight.

Usually if glucose and ketones appear together it indicates poor diabetes control, although this may pass off quickly so that glucose and ketones, present in the morning, may disappear by noon. If they are both a permanent feature, your diabetes needs to be better controlled, probably by increasing the insulin dose.

On rare occasions, ketones may appear in the urine without glucose. This is most likely to be found in the first morning specimen and probably occurs because the insulin taken the previous night is wearing off. Under these circumstances it is not serious and no action is needed.

Finally, ketones without glucose in the urine are very common in people who are trying to lose weight through calorie restriction. Anyone on a strict diet and losing weight will burn up body fat, which causes ketones to appear in the urine. Provided that there is no excess glucose in your urine, these ketones are of no concern and probably indicate that you are losing weight by breaking down body fat.

For some time now I have suffered from diabetes. Can you tell me what type of tests are made on my urine specimens when they are taken off to the laboratory?

Urine specimens are tested for several things but the most common are glucose, ketones and albumin (protein). These tests serve only as a spot check and are meant to complement your own tests performed at home. Clinics still tend to test the percentage of glucose in urine samples, even though the HbA_{1c} is a much better guide to diabetes control. The detection of ketones is of rather limited value since some people make ketones very easily and others almost not at all, but the presence of large amounts of ketones together with 2% glucose shows that the diabetes is very badly out of control.

The presence of protein in the urine can indicate either infection in the urine or the presence of some kidney disease, which in people with diabetes is likely to be diabetic nephropathy, a long-term complication (see Chapter 9). A more recent test is for microalbuminuria; the test detects microscopic amounts of albumin in the urine and can show signs of very early kidney damage.

I have a strong family history of diabetes. My daughter recently tested her urine and found 2% glucose. However, her blood glucose was only 8 mmol/L. She underwent a glucose tolerance test and this was normal. Could she have diabetes or could there be another reason why she is passing glucose in her water?

It is very unlikely that she has diabetes if a glucose tolerance test was normal. If she had glucose in her urine during the glucose tolerance test when all the blood glucose readings were strictly normal, then this would indicate that she has a low renal threshold for glucose (as discussed at the beginning of this section). If this is the correct diagnosis, it is important to find out whether she passes glucose in her urine first thing in the morning while fasting or only after she has eaten. People who pass glucose in their urine during the fasting state do not have an increased incidence of development of diabetes, and the condition (called renal glycosuria) is inherited. If, on the other hand, your daughter passes glucose in the urine only after meals containing starch and sugar, this condition sometimes progresses to diabetes.

HAEMOGLOBIN A$_{1c}$

When I last went to the clinic, I had a test for haemoglobin A1c. What is this for and what are the normal values?

Haemoglobin A$_{1c}$ is a component of the red pigment of blood (haemoglobin A, or HbA) which carries oxygen from the lungs to the various organs in the body. The HbA$_{1c}$ is calculated as a percentage of total haemoglobin and can be measured by a variety of laboratory methods. HbA$_{1c}$ consists of HbA combined with glucose by a chemical link. The amount of HbA$_{1c}$ present is directly proportional to the average blood glucose during the 120-day life span of the HbA-containing red blood corpuscles in the circulating blood.

HbA$_{1c}$ is the standard test for assessing long term diabetes control. Blood glucose levels fluctuate widely in the course of the day in people with Type 1 diabetes. Thus a single blood sugar measurement does not provide much information about overall control. HbA$_{1c}$ averages out the peaks and troughs of the blood glucose over the previous two to three months. Normal values vary a little from one laboratory to another and this can be a source of confusion as results from different clinics cannot be compared directly. Diabetes UK is trying to correct this anomaly by standardising methods used to measure HbA$_{1c}$. Normal values usually run between 4.5% and 6.1% but you must check the normal range in your local laboratory. Someone with poorly controlled diabetes may have an HbA$_{1c}$ as high as 15%, which reflects a consistently raised blood glucose over the previous couple of months. People with newly diagnosed diabetes normally have very high HbA$_{1c}$ levels until the treatment takes effect.

On the other hand someone with perfect control will have an HbA_{1c} around the upper end of the normal range – usually about 6%. An HbA_{1c} below 6% may indicate unrecognised hypos.

I've just had a fructosamine test but I didn't like to ask what this was for. What is this test?

The fructosamine test is similar to HbA_{1c} and indicates the average level of blood glucose over a shorter period of time – approximately two to three weeks. It measures the amount of glucose linked to proteins in the blood; the higher the blood glucose concentration, the higher the fructosamine. It has the advantage of being quicker and cheaper for the laboratory to measure but the disadvantage is that it is not as reliable and reproducible. The normal values may vary from one laboratory to another depending on the way the analysis is performed; in general a value less than 300 micromoles/litre is normal. In order to make sure you don't get confused, we suggest you pay particular attention to what is done in your clinic; don't hesitate to ask for a clear explanation.

I am 25 years old and have had diabetes since I was 15. I have been attending the clinic regularly every three months and do regular blood glucose tests at home with my own meter. At my last clinic visit, the doctor I saw said that he did not need to see me again for a whole year because my HbA_{1c} was consistently normal – why did he do this?

It sounds as though your specialist has great confidence in your ability to control your diabetes. As long as you can keep it this way, he clearly feels that seeing you once a year is sufficient. He can then spend more time with other people who are not as successful as you are. On the other hand, if you find the clinic visits helpful and motivating, it may be disappointing to be left 'on your own' for so long. You could try arranging to see the doctor or practice nurse at your surgery. They may provide the support you need.

My recent HbA$_{1c}$ was said to be low at 6%. Blood glucose readings look all right, on average about 5 mmol/litre. The specialist asked me to set the alarm clock and check them at 3 a.m. – why is this?

A low HbA$_{1c}$ suggests that at some stage your blood glucose levels are running unduly low. If you are not having hypoglycaemic attacks during the day, then it is possible that they are occurring at night and you are sleeping through them. By doing 3 a.m. blood glucose tests you should be able to determine whether this is so. Incidentally, you will only have to do these middle-of-the-night tests until you have established whether or not you are having hypos at night – they are not going to be a permanent part of your routine!

DIABETES CLINICS

My GP is starting a diabetes clinic in the local group practice and tells me that I no longer need to attend the hospital clinic. It's much more convenient for me to go to see my GP but will this be all right?

You are fortunate that your general practitioner has a special interest in diabetes and has gone to the trouble of setting up a special clinic in the practice for this. Many GPs and practice nurses have had special training in diabetes and these general practice-based diabetes clinics are becoming more common. They usually work well as long as you have uncomplicated diabetes and are well controlled, but you should be aware of the sort of care you can expect: Diabetes UK's recommendations are given in Figure 4.2. We are sure that your hospital specialist will know about your GP's new clinic and may even attend it from time to time. If you have any anxieties, why not discuss them with your doctor?

My GP is keen to test my urine every year to 'look for evidence of kidney damage'. This sounds very frightening. Please explain.

The test goes by the name of microalbuminuria. For years nurses in diabetic clinics have asked for a urine sample which they test for protein. This is a crude test and is only positive when there is a lot of protein in the urine. The new test is very sensitive and detects minute traces of albumin (the body's most common protein). Research has shown that protein detected in such small amounts is the first sign of kidney damage but at this early stage it can be reversed. This damage can be slowed by keeping the blood pressure below 135/75 and controlling the blood glucose – HbA_{1c} 7% or less. The result of this test is often presented as a ratio of albumin (the protein) to creatinine, which corrects for the flow of urine at the time. The best result is to have a ratio of less than 0.5. The top limit of normal is usually quoted as 3.5 for women and 2.5 for men. If left untreated, the amount of protein in the urine will increase until it can be detected by conventional urine testing sticks. Over a period of years, this may progress to kidney failure and the possible need for dialysis or a kidney transplant. At the early stage of microalbuminuria, this process is reversible by control of blood pressure and glucose. There is good evidence that people with normal blood pressure and microalbuminuria can be protected by treatment with a tablet called an ACE inhibitor.

I have had diabetes for ten years and used to be seen in the hospital clinic once a year. Now my practice nurse has asked me to see her every three months. Is there an explanation?

When diabetes was regarded as a 'hospital condition', the clinics tended to be enormous and because of pressure of numbers, people were normally seen every 6 or 12 months. It is universally agreed that everyone with diabetes should have an annual series of checks – known as the annual review – so the maximum time between appointments should be 12 months (see *What care to expect* in Figure 4.2). When the results of the UKPDS and DCCT trials demonstrated the importance of good control in preventing complications, it became clear that regular contact with healthcare professionals was necessary to achieve and maintain tight control. People in these studies were seen every three months. Many primary care clinics see people with diabetes every three to six months – or more frequently if there is a specific problem to be solved. It is important to have regular, structured diabetes care and the time between visits should be agreed between you and the doctor or nurse.

> *At my clinic we have a mixture of people ranging from young children to very old pensioners – why do they not have special clinics for young people?*

The NSF has specific standards for young people with diabetes (see p. 124). These include clear arrangements for transition from the children's clinic to the adult clinic. Most hospital clinics have special arrangements for young adults with diabetes so their particular needs can be addressed and it should not be necessary for young people to attend the same clinic as older people. Young people with diabetes have special needs, which are not usually met by an ordinary diabetes clinic. Growing up and learning to be independent places extra strains on diabetes control and young people prefer a more informal approach from members of the diabetes team. Some hospitals find it difficult to make these changes and there may be extra costs. However, clinics for young people have been set up in many parts of the country and you could ask your GP if you could be referred to one of them.

> *As a newly diagnosed person with diabetes what sort of care should I expect?*

Diabetes UK issued a document in June 2000 called *What diabetes care to expect*. This has been updated recently but the basics haven't changed. The list should probably include a routine test for microalbuminuria – see the question above in this section. This document explains clearly what standards of care to expect and some of the guidelines from it are reproduced in Figure 4.2. If you would like a copy of the complete document, contact Diabetes UK (address in Appendix 2).

I've had Type 1 diabetes for more than 30 years and throughout this time have been to the hospital diabetic clinic twice a year. I've now been told that I can no longer be seen at the hospital and that I must see my GP instead. As you can imagine, I am feeling rather anxious about this. What is the reason for the change?

We can understand your anxiety and will try to provide the reassurance you need, though of course that is difficult without knowing your local situation. The government is committed to altering the balance of diabetes care so that most of it is now carried out in GP surgeries. This has required additional education and many practice nurses and GPs have taken extra academic qualifications in diabetes. At the start of this process, GPs took on people with Type 2 diabetes who were controlled by diet or tablets or both. Once they needed insulin, people would be referred to the hospital clinic or diabetes specialist nurses, who would initiate insulin treatment. Such people would often continue to come to the hospital indefinitely. Now, the majority of health centres have gained confidence and experience in the use of insulin, and many GPs and practice nurses are also able to take on the care of people with Type 1 diabetes.

People with diabetes who have complex associated medical problems will probably continue to come to hospital clinics but so far no clear cut-off points have been defined.

Figure 4.2 What diabetes care to expect

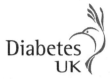

Diabetes
UK

WHAT CARE TO EXPECT FROM YOUR HEALTHCARE TEAM

Whether you have just been diagnosed or had diabetes for some time it is important that you get regular high quality healthcare. This will help to ensure that your diabetes, blood pressure and blood fats are all kept in check as well as detecting any early signs of complications so that they can be caught and treated successfully.

To achieve the best possible diabetes care, you need to work together with healthcare professionals as equal members of your diabetes care team. It is essential that you understand your diabetes as well as possible so that you are an effective member of this team.

You need to discuss with your consultant or GP the roles and responsibilities of those providing your diabetes care and to identify the key members of your own diabetes care team.

MEMBERS OF YOUR HEALTHCARE TEAM

- yourself
- consultant physician/diabetologist
- GP
- practice nurse
- dietitian
- optometrist/ophthalmologist
- podiatrist/chiropodist

- psychologist
- other medical specialists
- pharmacist

You may see some members of your diabetes care team more often than others.

WHEN YOU HAVE JUST BEEN DIAGNOSED

When you have just been diagnosed, your diabetes care team should:

- Give you a full medical examination.

- Work with you to make a programme of care which suits you and includes diabetes management goals – this may take the form of a record for you to keep.

- Arrange for you to talk with a diabetes specialist nurse (or practice nurse) who will explain what diabetes is and discuss your individual treatment and the equipment you will need to use.

- Arrange for you to talk with a state registered dietitian, who will want to know what you usually eat, and will give you advice on how to fit your usual diet in with your diabetes – a follow-up meeting should be arranged for more detailed advice.

- Tell you about your diabetes and the beneficial effects of a healthy diet, exercise and good diabetes control.

- Discuss the effects of diabetes on your job, driving, insurance, prescription charges, and if you are a driver, whether you need to inform the DVLA and your insurance company.

- Provide you with regular and appropriate information and education, on food and footcare for example.

- Give you information about Diabetes UK services and details of your local Diabetes UK voluntary group.

Figure 4.2 (*continued*)

WHEN YOUR DIABETES IS REASONABLY CONTROLLED

Once your diabetes is reasonably controlled, you should:

- Have access to your diabetes care team at least once a year – in this session, take the opportunity to discuss how your diabetes affects you as well as your diabetes control.

- Be able to contact any member of your diabetes care team for specialist advice, in person or by phone.

- Have further education sessions when you are ready for them.

- Have a formal medical annual review once a year with a doctor experienced in diabetes.

ON A REGULAR BASIS

On a regular basis, your diabetes care team should:

- Provide continuity of care, ideally from the same doctors and nurses – if this is not possible , the doctors or nurses who you are seeing should be fully aware of your medical history and background.

- Work with you to continually review your care programme, including your diabetes management goals.

- Let you share in decisions about your treatment or care.

- Let you manage your own diabetes in hospital after discussion with your doctor, if you are well enough to do so and that is what you wish.

- Organise pre- and post-pregnancy advice, together with an obstetric hospital team, if you are planning to become, or already are, pregnant.

- Encourage a carer to visit with you, to keep them up to date on diabetes so that they can make informed judgements about diabetes care.

- Encourage the support of friends, partners and/or relatives.
- Provide you with education sessions and appointments if you wish.
- Give you advice on the effects of diabetes and its treatments when you are ill or taking other medication.

WITH YOUR TREATMENT

If you are treated by insulin injections you should:

- Have frequent visits showing how to inject, look after your insulin and syringes and dispose of sharps (needles). You should also be shown how to test your blood glucose and test for ketones and be informed what the results mean and what to do about them.
- Be given supplies of, or a prescription for the medication and equipment you need.
- Discuss hypoglycaemia (hypos): when and why they may happen and how to deal with them.

If you are treated by tablets you should:

- Be given instruction on blood or urine testing and have explained what the results mean and what to do about them.
- Be given supplies of, or a prescription for the medication and equipment you need.
- Discuss hypoglycaemia (hypos): when and why they may happen and how to deal with them.

If you are treated by diet alone you should:

- Be given instruction on blood or urine testing and have explained what the results mean and what to do about them.
- Be given supplies of equipment you may need.

I've heard a lot of talk about the Diabetes NSF. What is it and how will it affect me?

Several years ago the Department of Health set up a scheme called the National Service Framework (NSF), which set out standards of care for a number of long-term conditions, such as heart disease and mental health. Diabetes was chosen as an important condition for which clear standards of care were needed.

The first section of the Diabetes NSF was published in 2001. This contained the agreed Standards of Care and was followed by the Delivery Strategy, which was published in 2003. This was designed to be implemented over several years with all targets achieved by 2013. The first target to be met was screening for retinopathy by digital photography to be available for all people with diabetes by the end of 2007.

The NSF Standards are printed in this chapter. The Delivery Strategy is a 40-page document which lacks a summary. However, it contains some worthy aspirations and we hope there will be funding to make these a reality. The NSF website: www.dh.gov.uk/PolicyAndGuidance/ HealthAndSocialCareTopics/Diabetes has the document.

The key elements proposed in this *Delivery Strategy* are:

- setting up a local diabetes network, or similar robust mechanism, which involves identifying local leaders and appointing and resourcing network managers, clinical champions and a person(s) with diabetes to champion the views of local people

- reviewing the local baseline assessment, establishing and promulgating local implementation arrangements with a trajectory to reach the standards

- participating in comparative local and national audit

- undertaking a local workforce skills profile of staff involved in the care of people with diabetes and developing education and training programmes with the local Workforce Development Confederation.

It also reflects targets in *Improvement, Expansion and Reform: the next three years*:

- ensuring a systematic eye-screening programme to national standards
- putting in place registers, education and advice, to support systematic treatment regimens.

The *Delivery Strategy* offers a framework for the NHS to build capacity to:

- put in place building blocks for the NHS to reach the National Service Framework (NSF) standards over the next ten years
- deliver the national targets.

I've been told my GP will be paid extra if my HbA$_{1c}$ is less that 7.5%. Can this be true?

This may sound a bit surprising, but it is true that the government has recently changed the way GPs are paid by negotiating a new contract based partly on the level of care achieved. For many conditions there is evidence that if certain targets are reached, the outcome is greatly improved. Thus, we know that for people with diabetes the risk of complications is significantly reduced if the HbA$_{1c}$ is less than 7.5%. Similarly, a blood pressure of less than 140/80 and a cholesterol of less than 4 mmol/L will reduce the risk of heart attack and stroke. The government believes that providing GPs with incentives to achieve these targets will drive up standards of care. The early signs are that this strategy has had some success.

My GP and practice nurse are putting pressure on me to improve control of my diabetes. I have heard that this is because they will be paid more if I get my HbA$_{1c}$ down to 7.4%. Why should I do this just to increase my doctor's income?

Although you may feel that lowering your HbA$_{1c}$ is more for your doctor's benefit than yours, it is important to remember that the reason the government introduced these targets for GPs is that there is strong evidence to show that people with diabetes have fewer health problems if their HbA_{1c} is less then 7.5%. Thus, it is in your own interests to improve the control of your diabetes. It is sad that the targets, introduced as a way of improving care for people with diabetes, have altered the doctor–patient relationship and given some people the impression that their doctor is more concerned about income than patient care.

BRITTLE DIABETES

What is brittle diabetes and what treatment does it require?

The term 'brittle diabetes' is used when the blood glucose of some- one with Type 1 diabetes oscillates from one extreme to another, with swings from severe hyperglycaemia (much too high) to severe hypoglycaemia (much too low). Many people taking insulin experi- ence blood glucose swings from time to time and the term 'brittle diabetes' is therefore restricted to those cases where the erratic blood glucose levels cause repeated admission to hospital.

Brittle diabetes is not a special type of diabetes and the term only applies when the instability is severe. This often occurs during peri- ods of stress or emotional uncertainty and it is particularly common amongst teenagers. Brittle diabetes often improves with time, usually when circumstances change, and it is unusual for it to persist indefinitely. There is no specific treatment but people with this condi- tion benefit from increased support from friends and family and from the diabetes team.

I have 'brittle diabetes' and my doctor has advised me to stop working. Am I entitled to any benefits?

The term 'brittle diabetes' is often used rather too loosely. The strict definition is when the blood glucose rises and falls very quickly, requiring frequent admission to hospital. Many conditions may contribute to this, including irregular meals and lifestyle, poor injection technique and lack of understanding of how to balance food, exercise and insulin. Few people find controlling their diabetes is so difficult that they have to give up work, but state benefits are available to people with diabetes in the same way as they are to anyone else. There are some questions about Social Security benefits in Chapter 5.

5 | Life with diabetes

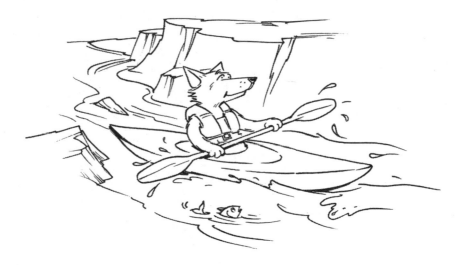

This chapter attempts to answer all the questions about issues that affect daily living when you have diabetes. It covers a broad sweep ranging from sport and holidays to surgical operations and illness. The section *Other illnesses* should be read early on, so that you will know how to react if you are struck down by a bad attack of flu. All car drivers should read the section *Driving*. At the end of the chapter is a miscellaneous section on issues which did not fall into the main sections: questions on electrolysis, ear piercing and identity bracelets for example. After reading this chapter, you will realise that there are very few activities that are barred to people with diabetes. Provided that you understand the condition, you should be able to do almost anything you wish.

SPORTS

My 13-year-old son is a keen footballer and has just developed diabetes. Will he be able to continue football and other sports? If so, what precautions should he take?

Your son can certainly keep on with his football. Well known professional footballers have played at an international level with Type 1 diabctes so, if your son is good enough, diabetes should not stop him getting to the top. People with diabetes have excelled in other sports, such as rugby, cricket, tennis, sailing, rowing, orienteering and mountaineering. Certainly all normal school sports should be encouraged.

There is, of course, the difficulty that the extra energy used in competitive sports increases the risk of a hypo. Your son should take some extra carbohydrate *before* a match or any other sports period – he could have a couple of sandwiches or biscuits or Jaffa cakes. He could also reduce his insulin dose at the meal before he takes exercise. He may nced another snack or a sugary drink like fruit juice or Lucozade® at half-time, and if possible should carry glucose tablets in his pocket.

He also needs to watch what he eats *after* the game. The effect of exercise on the body can last well after the exercise has stopped (the muscles are restocking their energy stores by converting glucose into glycogen). The blood glucose may drop two or more hours after the exercise period, so he may need a snack at that time. If he is due a meal anyway, he may need to eat more than usual. It would also be a good idea to increase the usual bedtime snack if he has been exercising in the afternoon or evening. It's always best to monitor blood glucose levels frequently in this situation.

*I used to enjoy swimming, but have been worried about going
back to the pool since I have been on insulin. What if I had a
hypo?*

While a hypo during athletics and most team games can be
inconvenient, a hypo while swimming can be more serious
and you are right to be concerned about it. However, don't let your
concern stop you swimming. There are certain simple rules that all
people taking insulin should follow before swimming; these will
allow you to swim with complete safety.

- Never swim alone.

- Tell your companions (or teacher if you are still at school) to
  pull you out of the water if you behave oddly or are in
  difficulty.

- Check your blood glucose before swimming and take some
  Lucozade® (or equivalent) if it is less than 8 mmol/L.

- Keep glucose tablets or Lucozade® on the side of the pool.

- Get out of the water immediately at the first signs of a hypo.

If you are a keen swimmer and want to take up scuba diving, the
British Sub-Aqua Club does impose some restrictions. It requires
people taking insulin who wish to scuba dive to have an annual
medical review, to be free of any long-term complications of
diabetes, and insist that they always dive with another person who
does not have diabetes. You can contact the Club for more details –
the address is in Appendix 2.

Can I take part in all or any forms of sport?

The vast majority of sports are perfectly safe for people with
diabetes. The problem lies in those sports where loss of control
due to a hypo could be dangerous, not only to you but to fellow

participants or spectators. Swimming is an example of a potentially dangerous sport but, if you take certain precautions, it is safe (see previous question). However, in some sports (such as motor racing) the risk of serious injury in the case of a hypo is even greater. The governing bodies of such high-risk sports discourage people with diabetes from taking part. Discouragement does not necessarily mean a total ban – the restrictions may vary depending on your treatment. You can always contact the appropriate governing body to ask what (if any) restrictions they impose. Skiing is discussed in the section *Holidays and travel* later in this chapter.

Are people with diabetes allowed to go parachuting? I want to do a sponsored parachute jump to raise money for charity.

You can probably do your sponsored jump but there are some restrictions for people taking insulin. You will need a medical certificate to state that you are well controlled, and you will be permitted to jump only in tandem. The British Parachute Association (address in Appendix 2) can give you more information about this.

As a 30-year-old with diabetes, can I join a keep fit class or do a work-out at home?

Keeping fit is important for everybody. Like everyone else, if you are unused to exercise, you should build up the exercises slowly week by week to avoid damaging muscles or tendons. Remember that exercise usually has the effect of lowering blood glucose, so you may need to reduce the insulin dose or take extra carbohydrate beforehand (see the first question in this section).

I take insulin and jog quite a bit. I would like to try running a marathon. Have you any advice on the subject?

Dawn Kenwright, who has Type 1 diabetes, has many years of experience of running at international level. She resumed training within weeks of starting insulin and worked hard to discover by trial and error the effect of exercise, food and insulin on her blood glucose levels. Before running, Dawn has found that she needs plenty of 'slow' carbohydrate (in the form of porridge) to maintain her energy levels. During training sessions Dawn wears a bumbag containing glucose tablets and solution, but in competition she cuts back her insulin drastically and just carries glucose tablets. With careful preparation she rarely needs extra glucose. Dawn warns you to progress gradually from jogging up to a full marathon distance. She stresses that what is right for her will not necessarily suit everyone and makes the point that each athlete with diabetes has to work out their own solution for their particular sport.

Diabetes UK produces factsheets on long-distance running and some other sports. Once you have reached the required standard, you should think of joining Diabetes UK's team for the London Marathon.

EATING OUT

My wife and I entertain a great deal and we often go out for meals in a restaurant. I have recently been diagnosed with Type 1 diabetes. How am I going to cope with eating out, now I am on insulin?

Nowadays people with diabetes usually eat similar food to anyone who is following a healthy lifestyle. Although you should normally try to avoid foods that are obviously high in sugar and fat, this may be difficult when you are visiting friends.

Restaurants or takeaways should pose less of a problem as you can select suitable dishes from the menu. Many people using a basal bolus regimen choose to take additional short-acting insulin to cover the extra food they are eating. Estimating the amount of carbohydrate in the food and deciding how much insulin you need is a skill which develops with experience. In an earlier section (see p. 91) we have talked about the DAFNE method, which teaches you how to calculate your insulin dose accurately. If you are uncertain about the size of portion you will be given in a restaurant you should wait until you see what is on your plate before deciding on the dose of insulin.

Sometimes people worry about how they are going to give their injections when they are away from home. With an insulin pen there should be no difficulty and most people are able to give the insulin discreetly at the table when the food arrives. Do not take your evening dose of insulin before leaving home in case the meal is delayed.

FASTING AND DIABETES

As a Muslim I wish to fast during Ramadan. Is this possible?

People with diabetes who fast during Ramadan may experience large swings in blood glucose levels, as a result of the long gaps between meals and the consumption of large quantities of carbohydrate-rich foods during the non-fasting hours. Therefore, if you have diabetes, you may be exempt from fasting. However, many people with diabetes do not want to be exempted from a religious observance that they feel strongly about. If you are taking twice-daily insulin, it will be very difficult to go for long periods without eating. If you take basal bolus insulin, provided you take your background insulin in the usual way, you should be able to change the timing and dose of your meal time insulin to fit in with the Ramadan eating pattern.

My local youth group is holding a sponsored fast over a weekend. I have Type 1 diabetes – can I take part?

It would be very difficult and perhaps dangerous for you to go without food and, even more important, drink, for 48 hours. The problem is that, even in the fasting state, you need small amounts of insulin to prevent the blood glucose rising. Having taken insulin, you would then need food to prevent an overshoot leading to a hypo. Anyone who goes without food for long periods produces ketones, which could be another hazard. Can you think of anything else you could do to raise money while your friends are fasting?

HOLIDAYS AND TRAVEL

Do you have any simple rules for people with diabetes going abroad for holidays?

Here is a checklist of things to take with you (in your hand luggage).

- Insulin
- Syringes or insulin pen and needles
- Test strips, meter, finger pricker and lancets
- Glucose tablets
- Glucogel® (Hypostop)
- Glucagon
- Starchy carbohydrate in case meals are delayed
- Other prescribed medications (keep a list)
- Identification bracelet, necklace or card
- Medical insurance

- European Health Insurance Card (EHIC), which has replaced Form E111 if travelling inside EU (see question on p. 140)

- Letter from your doctor confirming that you need to carry equipment for injections and blood testing

Is it safe for someone with diabetes to take travel sickness tablets?

Travel sickness pills do not upset diabetes, although they may make you sleepy so be careful if you are driving. On the other hand, vomiting can upset diabetes so it is worthwhile trying to avoid travel sickness. If you do become sick, the usual rules apply. Continue to take your normal dose of insulin and take carbohydrate in some palatable liquid form, such as a sugary drink. Test your blood glucose regularly.

Each year on our summer holidays, our daughter becomes violently sick on the ferry. She recovers quite soon after we get back on dry land but she can keep nothing down during the crossing and it is very worrying.

We presume your daughter is on insulin and, as a general rule, people on insulin need hospital help once they start vomiting. Profuse vomiting leads to dehydration and if this is severe, the only treatment is a 'drip'. The other worry is the risk of a hypo if your daughter has already had her insulin. Don't be tempted to stop her insulin on the grounds that she is not eating.

There is no simple solution (apart from going by the Channel Tunnel) but the following ground rules may help.

- Take a standard anti-sickness tablet (e.g. Sea-legs®) at the recommended time before you sail.

- Try the 'acupressure' wrist bands for seasickness now on sale at most chemists.

- Do frequent blood tests during the journey and immediately afterwards.

- If she has basal bolus insulin, you should still give background (basal) insulin.

- If her blood glucose rises alarmingly, try giving her extra small doses of short-acting insulin.

- If her blood glucose values fall too low, give her Lucozade®, or some other non-diet soft drink.

We are going on holiday and wish to take a supply of insulin and glucagon with us. How should I store them both for the journey and in the hotel?

Insulin is very stable and will keep for one month at room temperature in our temperate climate. However, it does not like extremes of temperature and can be damaged if kept too long at high temperatures or if frozen. It is best to carry your supplies in more than one piece of luggage in case one suitcase goes astray.

If you are travelling by air you should keep your insulin in your hand luggage – temperatures in the luggage hold of an aircraft usually fall below freezing and insulin left in luggage there could be damaged. Insulin manufacturers say it is stable for one month at 25°C (77°F), so it is perfectly safe to keep insulin with your luggage on the average holiday. Avoid the glove compartment or the boot of your car where very high temperatures can be reached. In tropical conditions your stock of insulin should be kept in the fridge.

Storage of glucagon is no problem as this comes as a powder with a vial of water for dilution. It is very stable and can survive extremes of heat and cold.

In these days of increased airport security, people traveling with normal equipment needed to manage their diabetes are being challenged for evidence that their materials are bona fide, which can be extremely irritating. Security staff need to see a list on official (hospital or GP practice) headed notepaper of the items to be carried. Alternatively you can obtain an insulin user's identification card online or by phone from Diabetes UK at a cost of £5. Also available from Diabetes UK is a treatment identity card for £1.50.

I would like to go on a skiing holiday. Is it safe for me to ski, skate and toboggan? Should I take special precautions?

It is as safe for someone with diabetes to ski and enjoy other winter sports as it is for anyone else. Accidents do occur and it is essential to take out adequate insurance to cover all medical expenses. Read the small print in the insurance form carefully to ensure that it does not exclude pre-existing conditions like diabetes, or require them to be declared. In this case you should contact the insurance company and if necessary take out extra medical cover for your diabetes. Diabetes UK can provide travel insurance that will cover your diabetes (see Appendix 2). Physical activity increases the likelihood of hypos so always carry glucose and a snack as you may be delayed, especially if you are injured. Never go without a sensible companion who knows you have diabetes and understands what to do if you have a hypo.

Do make sure your ski boots are properly fitted, particularly if you have any degree of neuropathy. Poorly fitting boots are a very common cause of foot damage and ulceration.

Is sunbathing all right for people with diabetes?

Of course people with diabetes can sunbathe. Lying around doing nothing may put your blood glucose up a little, especially if you overeat as most people do on holiday. So keep up your usual tests as you may need extra insulin. On the other hand, increasing the temperature of the skin may speed up the absorption of the insulin and can lead to hypos, so be prepared for changes. Remember that sunbathing can increase the risk of skin cancer whether or not you have diabetes, so always take sensible precautions to avoid sunburn by covering up, in the middle of the day particularly, and using sun-screen with a high protection factor.

As I have diabetes should I be vaccinated when going abroad?

People with diabetes should have exactly the same vaccinations as anyone else. You are no more or less likely to contract illnesses abroad but, if you do become ill, the consequences could be more serious. In addition to the necessary vaccinations, it is very important to take protective tablets against malaria if you are going to a tropical area where this disease is found. More cases of this potentially serious disease are being seen in this country, usually in travellers recently returned from Africa or the Far East.

I am going to work in the Middle East for six months. What can I do if my insulin is not available in the country where I am working?

If you are working abroad for six months only, it should be quite easy to take enough insulin to last you this length of time. Stored in an ordinary fridge it should keep – but make sure that you are not supplied with insulin near the end of its shelf life. The expiry date is printed on each box of insulin.

Most types of insulin are available in the Middle East, but you may have to make do with a different brand name or even insulin from a different source (pig, cow or human). Porcine insulin may be hard to obtain in strict Muslim countries. U100 (100 units/mL) insulin may be difficult to obtain outside the UK, USA, Australia, New Zealand and South Africa. Some contries in Europe, parts of the Far East and South America may only stock insulin in 40 units/mL (U40) and you will have to obtain special syringes for use with U40 insulin. Diabetes UK can tell you which insulin strength is used in the country you are going to.

If you are using an insulin pen – either disposable or the cartridge variety – it would be better to take all your insulin requirements with you as it may be difficult to obtain the pens or cartridges you need. Remember to take a spare pen.

> *My partner has just been offered an excellent post in Uruguay, which he would love to accept. He is worried about my diabetes there and especially about the availability of my insulin. Can you let me know if my insulin can be sent by post?*

It should be possible to obtain an equivalent type of insulin to your own in most parts of the world. If you are keen to keep up your normal supplies, Hypoguard Ltd will despatch syringes and equipment for testing blood and urine to all parts of the world. Unfortunately Hypoguard is not able to handle insulin. You might be able to make arrangements with a high street chemist who would be prepared to send insulin by post. John Bell & Croyden in London will send insulin abroad. The address is in Appendix 2.

> *My friends and I are going to Spain to work next year. Can you tell me what I should take with me and whether I would have to pay if I needed to see a doctor?*

It is now common for people from the UK to live in other European countries for long periods, if not for good. Generally speaking, professional diabetes care is excellent in the fully developed countries and you should expect the same process of screening for complications and help with diabetes as in the UK. Before you go abroad, you should ask your doctor for a full report of your medical condition. This should include the following:

- Details of insulin and method of injecting (e.g. type of penfill);
- Name of blood glucose testing strips;
- Recent blood pressure measurement;
- All other medication – using official rather than brand names, e.g. ramipril rather than Tritace®;

- Results of recent blood tests (HbA_{1c}, creatinine, cholesterol);

- Microalbuminuria test result;

- Latest retinal screening result – if any abnormalities, try to obtain a digital record of the photographs by email or on CD;

- Results of latest foot screening;

- Details of any known complications of diabetes.

Before you go abroad prepare well: take spares of insulin pens, testing equipment and so on, and keep spares separate from the main supply in case your luggage is lost.

Medical attention is free in all European Union countries, although you should obtain a European Health Insurance Card (EHIC) which replaces the old E111 certificate. You can order an EHIC online for £15. For longer stays abroad, you should contact the DSS. For countries outside the EU, you should insure your health before you go. Diabetes UK Careline can help you with this (see Chapter 11 for contact details).

I take insulin and need to fly to the USA. How do I cope with the changing time zones?

The most important advice when travelling long distance is to test your blood glucose more frequently than usual – at least every four to five hours. This may be inconvenient but travel is often unpredictable and curious things happen to diabetes control. The only way to keep safe is to test often, even if you're not normally a frequent tester. If you do have a bad hypo while aboard, the cabin crew will have to deal with it and they may not be particularly knowledgeable about diabetes.

If you take basal bolus insulin (short-acting insulin with each meal and long-acting insulin at bedtime) you should continue to take short-acting insulin each time you eat. If you take background (basal) insulin in two divided doses, it should be simple to swap round the morning and evening doses in the new time zone. However, if you only have a single daily injection of background insulin at bedtime, you need to decide whether or not to change the time you have this injection. If it is a short trip, you should continue to have background insulin at the same UK time as normal. However, if you are spending more than a week in the new time zone, it would be worth moving the time of the injection to bedtime. For instance, the East coast of USA is five hours behind UK time and you are likely to arrive in the afternoon, though your body clock will think it is five hours later. Provided you have short-acting insulin every four hours, you should be able to delay your background insulin till bedtime. If you are travelling in the opposite direction, the interval between long-acting injections will be shorter than usual so you may need to reduce the first dose of background insulin on arrival. If you underestimate the amount of insulin you need you can always correct with a small dose of short-acting insulin later. The key to the problem is frequent testing.

If you control your diabetes with an insulin pump, all you need to do is readjust the time clock.

I am on twice-daily mixtures of insulin and am flying to Los Angeles on holiday. How will the change in time affect my diabetes?

If your diabetes is not well controlled on your present insulin, this could be an opportunity to change to a more flexible insulin regime. However, if you are well controlled on premixed insulin, there are ways of adjusting your insulin to the conditions. It would be sensible to ask your GP for a supply of short-acting insulin (Humalog® or NovoRapid®) which you can take if your blood glucose starts to rise. Mixed insulin, which is mainly long-acting insulin, is not effective at reducing the blood glucose rapidly. The advice about blood testing (see previous question) applies and if at any time your glucose rises above 12 mmol/litre you should take insulin every four hours, preferably before a meal. The dose will depend on how much insulin you normally take in a day. Once you have arrived, continue to take short-acting insulin every four to six hours until you reach a time when you would normally take your premixed insulin – usually breakfast and evening meal. You can then go back to your normal insulin doses, though you must continue to test frequently as holidays are notorious for upsetting control of blood glucose. For specific advice, you should speak to your GP or diabetes specialist nurse.

Figure 5.1

TRAVEL TIPS

Flying across time zones can be confusing for anyone, and makes it difficult to know which meal you are eating. When travelling keep to the following rules.

- Do not aim at perfect control. You have to be flexible especially on international flights. A hypo while travelling can be very inconvenient.

- Be prepared to check your blood glucose if you are at all worried and unsure how much insulin you need.

- In general, airlines are prepared to make special allowances for people with diabetes and cabin crew will do their best to help. Airlines say that they like to be warned in advance.

- Most experienced travellers avoid special 'diabetic' meals which are usually very low in carbohydrate.

- Take two watches and keep one on UK time while you make the change in injection times. This will help you work out when you would be taking your insulin at home and you can then make gradual changes in injection times until you are synchronised with your new time zone.

WORK

Can I take a job involving shift work?

Many people combine shift work with good control of their blood glucose. Shift work does, however, demand a little extra care as most insulin regimens are designed round a 24-hour day. Shift workers usually complain that they are just settling into one routine when everything changes and they have to start again. It is hard to generalise about shift work as there are so many different patterns but, if you follow these rules, things should work out all right.

- Aim at an injection of short- and intermediate-acting insulin every 12–16 hours, or use a basal bolus regimen. This way of giving insulin makes it much simpler to plan for shift work.

- If you are taking twice-daily insulin you should eat carbohydrate at regular intervals while at work, just as you do when working normal daytime hours.

- If you take basal bolus insulin you should eat carbohydrate with every injection. It helps if you know how to count the carbohydrate so you can calculate how much insulin you need (see p. 101).

- If you take twice-daily insulin and need to delay your injections by more than six hours when you are changing from one shift to another, have some short-acting insulin on its own followed by a meal.

- Because your pattern of insulin and food is constantly changing, you will have to do more blood glucose measurements than normal, as you cannot assume that one day is very much like another.

- If your blood glucose results are not good, be prepared to make changes in your dose of insulin. You will soon become an expert about your own diabetes.

How can I cope with my diabetes if I work irregular hours as a sales rep?

Just as in shift work, many people manage to combine an irregular work pattern with good diabetes control. Those who lead an erratic lifestyle usually find that the basal bolus regimen gives them more freedom as it will allow them to miss or delay a meal without risk of a hypo. The basal bolus regimen is much easier to deliver using an insulin pen (see the section *Insulin pens* in Chapter 3).

If you take twice-daily insulin and have a normal blood glucose before lunch, you are likely to go hypo unless you eat at the right time. You will not be able to afford the luxury of missing meals completely but it is always possible to have a few biscuits or even a sweet drink if you are getting past your normal eating time.

The occupational hazard of all sales reps, with diabetes or otherwise, is the mileage that they clock up each year on the roads. With modern blood glucose meters, it should be possible to avoid the dangers of hypoglycaemia while driving.

The rules for driving are:

- Always check your blood glucose before driving;

- If it is low, eat or take a glucose drink before you drive;

- Always carry food in your car and have some immediately if you feel warning of a hypo;

- If you think you may be hypo, pull off the road immediately, stop the car, turn off the ignition and remove the key;

- Do not resume driving until you are sure your blood glucose is in the normal range.

Should I warn fellow employees that I might be subject to hypos?

It is never easy to give personal information to workmates, but unfortunately hypos do happen at work, especially when a person first starts using insulin. You should warn your workmates that, if they find you acting in a peculiar way, they must persuade you to take some sugar. Warn them also that you may not be very cooperative at the time and may even resist their attempts to help. It is difficult to admit to colleagues that you have diabetes but, if you keep it a secret, you run the risk of causing a scare by having a bad hypo. The natural response of your workmates will be to dial 999 and you may be taken to hospital by ambulance for treatment. You can probably avoid this worst-case scenario by giving your colleagues some useful diabetes education.

My partner's hours of work can be very erratic. Sometimes he only gets three or four hours' sleep instead of his normal eight hours. Can you tell me what effect lack of sleep has on diabetes?

Lack of sleep in itself will not affect diabetes although, if your partner is under great pressure, his blood glucose may be either higher or lower than usual. The real problem with working under a strain is the tendency to ignore diabetes completely and assume that it will look after itself. Unfortunately a few minutes of each day have to be spent checking blood glucose, eating a snack or giving insulin. These minutes are well spent.

I developed diabetes five months ago, one week after I had started a new job. I am coming to the end of my six-month probation period and have been given two weeks' notice because they say I cannot do shift work when I have diabetes. Can you help?

This is a sad story and a good example of ignorant prejudice against people with diabetes. Of course there are many people on shift work who maintain good control – although it does require a bit of extra thought. You may well have a case under the Disability Discrimination Act and you should seek advice from your local Citizen's Advice Bureau. If you are using the basal bolus insulin regime, there is no reason why you should not be able to adjust your insulin to your shifts. It may take a bit of juggling, but many people taking insulin manage in this way without any problem.

> *I am a pub manager and have had diabetes for the past 19 years but my employers are now making me redundant. Apparently, their insurers cannot accept me for a permanent position owing to my diabetes. Who can help strengthen my case?*

We know of several publicans with diabetes who successfully run pubs and still keep their diabetes under good control. However, people who work in licensed premises are at greater risk of drinking more alcohol than average, and heavy drinkers are in danger from hypos (see the section *Alcohol* later in this chapter). We wonder if you have been having frequent hypos, which has made it difficult to continue in your present occupation. Ask your doctor and Diabetes UK to lobby on your behalf and seek legal advice from your local Citizen's Advice Bureau.

> *I have been refused a job with a large company because of my diabetes. Have I sufficient grounds to take proceedings against them for discrimination?*

The Disability Discrimination Act covers people with diabetes but taking a company to court can be difficult. Unfortunately this sort of discrimination does happen, especially in large organisations, although it can be very difficult to prove. The support of your own diabetes team will be important if you wish to take proceedings under the Disability Discrimination Act.

Diabetes UK has had discussions with medical officers responsible for occupational health in several large organisations. There is useful information on the Diabetes UK website.

OTHER ILLNESSES

I have recently had a severe cough and cold and have been given 'diabetic' cough medicine by the doctor. Since then my blood glucose has been very high. Could this be due to the medicine?

Antibiotic syrup and cough linctus are often blamed for making diabetes worse during an illness such as flu or a chest infection. In fact a dose of antibiotic syrup only contains about 5 g of sugar and will have very little effect on your blood glucose. It is the illness itself that unbalances the diabetes. In general, medication from your doctor will not upset your diabetes.

Any infection or serious illness will cause a rise in blood glucose and it is important to test your blood if you feel unwell (see Chapter 12: **Emergencies**). You will probably need to increase your insulin dose during the illness and it is very important to continue regular insulin injections *even if you are not eating*. If you are vomiting and unable to keep fluids down, you will need hospital admission for intravenous fluids. Vomiting can sometimes be a sign of ketoacidosis, which may be fatal if untreated.

The rules for illness are:

- Test blood at least four times a day;

- If tests are high take extra doses of short-acting insulin;

- If the tests are low, take a sugary drink such as Lucozade® to treat the hypo;

- Never stop insulin.

It is of course possible to get over a bad cold by carrying on with your normal dose of insulin and accepting bad control for a few days. However, this means that your mouth and nose will be slightly dehydrated and it may take longer before you feel back to normal. You will probably feel better more quickly if you adjust your insulin and try to keep the blood glucose near normal.

I have noticed that my son suffers from more colds since developing diabetes. Could this be due to his diabetes?

Many parents make this observation, but there is no real reason why the common cold should be more common in diabetes. However, a relatively minor cold may upset his diabetes control and lead to several extra days of feeling unwell (see previous question). This may make it a more memorable event. To repeat the previous advice, never stop insulin.

My daughter keeps getting infections and has been rushed to hospital on several occasions with high ketones and requiring a drip. How can I prevent these infections? Will vitamins help?

It sounds as though your daughter has what is known as 'brittle diabetes' and this must be very alarming. Some people, particularly children, become very ill and 'sugary' at the first sniff of a cold or the beginning of an infection. In others, the problem may be that the blood glucose is running high most of the time and it doesn't take very much to push it up to a dangerous level. If your daughter's control is generally good, you will need to respond to any infection by testing her blood frequently and giving extra insulin if it is high (see Chapter 12: **Emergencies**). On the other hand if her blood sugar levels are usually high, we suggest you speak to the diabetes team to discuss what action to take.

My 6-year-old daughter who is on insulin is troubled with frequent vomiting that occurs suddenly. She has ended up in hospital on several occasions as she becomes dehydrated. What can I do to avoid this?

Vomiting in a young child with diabetes has to be taken seriously and admission to hospital is probably necessary to replace fluid losses by means of a drip.

High blood glucose levels and ketones lead to vomiting. It may be

LIFE WITH DIABETES | 149

possible to avoid the vomiting by giving extra short-acting insulin as soon as the blood glucose level rises. See Chapter 12: **Emergencies** or speak to your hospital diabetes team.

What is the best treatment for someone suffering from hay fever? I understand that some products can cause drowsiness, which could affect my balance and be confused with a hypo.

You can use exactly the same treatment for your hay fever as people without diabetes, as it does not affect your control. Antihistamines are often used for hay fever and these may make you feel sleepy, but this should be easy to distinguish from a hypo. Remember that, if you are on antihistamines, you should be very cautious about drinking alcohol. Hay fever can also be alleviated by using a nasal spray to reduce the sensitivity of the membranes in the nose.

I have just been in hospital with anaphylactic shock from a bee sting. I have diabetes and wondered if this had anything to do with the severity of my reaction?

There is no connection between diabetes and allergy to bees.

What is the effect of other illnesses on diabetes? Is my son likely to suffer more illness than other children of his age?

Any illness is likely to make the blood glucose rise and people on insulin need to increase the dose to keep this under control.

Diabetes itself does not necessarily make people prone to other illnesses. In fact a survey in a large American company revealed that people with diabetes had no more absences from work than those without. Most children with diabetes grow up without any more illness than their friends.

Type 1 diabetes is one of a group of conditions caused by the production of antibodies which have adverse effects on certain parts of

MORECAMBE BAY HOSPITALS NHS TRUST

the body. These may cluster in families and more than one condition may occur in a single individual. The most common conditions associated with Type 1 diabetes are thyroid disease (both over- and under-active) and coeliac disease.

> *Since I was diagnosed with Type 1 diabetes, I have been very depressed. Is there any link between depression and diabetes?*

The diagnosis of diabetes often comes as a great shock and people respond in different ways. Some are able to adjust to their new condition, while others find it very difficult to accept the impact it has on their lifestyle. They may experience a wide range of emotions which include anger, fear and grief over the loss of their good health. Later comes the harsh realisation that this is not a short-term condition and the energy required to meet the demands of diabetes has to be sustained for life. It is not surprising that many people become depressed when coping with these emotions and it can take time to work through this and adapt to the new situation.

Sometimes people combat these negative feelings by throwing themselves into activities such as sport with added enthusiasm and find their sense of achievement heightened by successfully overcoming the demands of diabetes.

> *I have heard that people with diabetes are more likely to be depressed. Is this true?*

This sounds like a simple question but it is not easy to answer. Many research studies have shown that the majority of people with diabetes have a normal quality of life, unless they are affected by complications which interfere with daily living. You would probably predict that a lifelong disease, which puts extra demands on people, would lead to depression, and it is probably about twice as common as in people without diabetes.

On the other hand, there are many people who already have a serious psychological disease such as depression, anxiety or an eating disorder, who then develop diabetes. Whatever the cause of their depression, people who feel negative about themselves cannot summon up the energy required to look after their diabetes and it is more difficult for them to achieve good control.

How does stress and worry affect diabetes? I spend many hours studying and find that, if I study too long, I feel weak and shaky. Are there any side effects to this sort of pressure that may affect my diabetes?

In general, stress and worry tend to increase the blood glucose. One student told us that in the run up to her final examination, she had to double her insulin dose to keep perfect blood glucose control, even though she did not appear to her friends to be particularly anxious. Stress causes a release of adrenaline and other hormones, which antagonise the effect of insulin.

During periods of stress it may be difficult to keep to strict mealtimes, so you could be at risk of going hypo. You should check your blood glucose and, if it is normal, you are simply experiencing the tiredness that we all feel after studying hard. Don't blame it on your diabetes but have an evening off from your studies.

HOSPITAL OPERATIONS

Recently, when I was in hospital to have my appendix removed, I was put on a 'sliding scale'. Please could you explain this, especially as it might save other people in a similar position from worrying?

The expression 'sliding scale' does sound rather alarming – but it is nothing to worry about. It can be difficult to predict exactly how much insulin someone will need during and after an operation, while they cannot eat or drink normally. The solution is to give glucose and insulin into a vein, with the dose of insulin adjusted depending on the blood glucose – known as a 'sliding scale'. More insulin is given if the level of blood glucose is high and this will have an immediate effect since it goes straight into the bloodstream. The blood glucose is usually checked every 1–2 hours and the insulin adjusted accordingly. In this way, diabetes control can be carefully regulated throughout the operation and until the person is eating again. Once this stage is reached, insulin may be given as three or four injections a day, the dose given at each injection being determined from the amount of insulin required during the 'sliding scale' period.

Are there any problems with surgery for a child with diabetes?

Surgical operations on children usually involve a general anaesthetic and it is advisable to have nothing to eat or drink ('nil by mouth') for six hours before the start of the anaesthetic. Any difficulties caused by this period of fasting can be overcome by a glucose drip into the vein. The normal insulin injection is not given on the day of operation but a small dose of insulin is normally pumped continuously into a vein. The dose of insulin is adjusted according to the blood glucose level. In minor operations where people are expected to be eating an hour or so later, these elaborate procedures may not be necessary and insulin may simply be delayed until the next meal is due.

If an emergency operation is necessary, it is important that the doctors know that your child has diabetes.

Must I tell my dentist that I have diabetes and will this affect my treatment in any way?

Having diabetes will not affect your dental treatment. However, it is important to remove all possibility of a hypo while you are in the dentist's chair. Warn your dentist that you cannot overrun a snack time or mealtime. It is less embarrassing to mention this before the start of a session than to have to munch glucose tablets while the dentist is trying to administer treatment. If your mouth is painful before or after your visit to the dentist, you may not be able to eat normal meals, which will require an adjustment in your insulin.

Obviously you must warn your dentist if you are due to have any form of heavy sedation. If someone on insulin is to have dental treatment needing a general anaesthetic, this is usually done in hospital.

Is someone with diabetes more likely to suffer from tooth decay or gum trouble?

There is an increased risk of infection in people whose diabetes is poorly controlled. The gums may become infected and this in turn may lead to tooth decay. However, someone who is well controlled is not prone to any particular dental problem – in fact, there is a positive advantage to avoiding sweets, which cause dental caries (tooth decay).

I have been told that, as I have diabetes, I don't have to pay for dental treatment. Is this true?

No. Dental treatment is not free to people who have diabetes. If you are entitled to benefits such as Income Support, you may be able to claim some help with the cost of treatment.

DRIVING

I drive a lot in my work and my lunchtime varies from day to day. Does this matter? I am on two injections of insulin a day.

This can be a problem. The twice-daily insulin regimen is designed to provide a boost of insulin at mid-day to cope with the lunchtime intake of food. Once the early morning injection of insulin has been given, there is no way of delaying the mid-day surge. It is very common for people who are well controlled on two injections a day to run a low blood sugar before lunch. Here are some possible solutions.

- Always check your blood glucose before driving, particularly if a meal is due. The DVLA now recommends this practice.

- Keep some food, such as biscuits or fruit, with you while driving so you can eat if your blood glucose goes low.

- Change to the basal bolus insulin regimen so that you have a small dose of short-acting insulin before each main meal with long-acting insulin in the evening to control your blood glucose overnight. If you use a rapid-acting analogue (such as NovoRapid® or Humalog®) you should not even need snacks between meals. However, we would still advise you to test before driving.

If I have diabetes, do I have to declare this when applying for a driving licence? If so, will I have to prove I am fit to drive?

Anyone on insulin treatment for diabetes must by law declare this to the DVLA (Drving and Vehicle Licensing Agency) when applying for a driving licence. If you already hold a driving licence, you must tell the DVLA as soon as you have been diagnosed.

When you have notified the DVLA, you will receive a form asking for details about your diabetes and the names of any doctors whom you see regularly. You will be asked to sign a declaration allowing your doctors to disclose medical details about your condition. There is usually no difficulty over someone with diabetes obtaining a licence to drive, though the bureaucracy may be irritating. The DVLA now advises people to test their blood glucose before driving, which is another cause of frustration but at least ensures that it is safe for you to drive.

You will be issued a licence valid for only three years instead of up to the age of 70, which is normal in the UK. It is the risk of sudden and severe hypoglycaemia which makes people liable to this form of discrimination. In general the only people who have difficulty in obtaining a licence are those with very erratic control and a history of hypos causing unconsciousness. Once their condition has been controlled and severe hypos abolished, they can reapply for a licence with confidence.

Diabetes UK has successfully campaigned for regulations on C1 licences to be changed. Previously, blanket restrictions were imposed on insulin users wishing to drive small vans and lorries of between 3.5 and 7.5 tonnes. The revised regulations enable anyone taking insulin to be individually assessed on their fitness to drive, even if they have previously had their entitlement withdrawn. Restrictions on other Group 2 vehicles (heavier vehicles and passenger-carrying vehicles, such as minibuses) remain. For more information, contact Diabetes UK.

When I was filling out a form for the DVLA, one of the questions asked whether I had had laser treatment in both eyes. Why do the DVLA need this information?

The DVLA may ask you to have a 'visual fields test' if you have had laser treatment in both eyes, and your licence will be revoked if you cannot pass this test. The reason behind this is that in a few cases, very heavy laser therapy can reduce the field of vision – making it like looking through a keyhole. If you are having a visual fields test, you should have the type in which both eyes are tested at the same time. This test is the DVLA driving standard.

Do I have to inform my insurance company that I have diabetes?

When applying for motor insurance, you must declare that you have diabetes. Failure to disclose this can invalidate your cover if you need to make a claim. The Disability Discrimination Act 1996 outlawed the charging of higher premiums for groups of people where no higher risk rate has been proven, as is the case with diabetes. Unfortunately, there are some companies that still discriminate, but Diabetes UK Services has arranged a car insurance scheme to help make life easier. (See Appendix 2 for more information.)

> *I have heard that a driver who had a motor accident while hypo was successfully prosecuted for driving under the influence of drugs and heavily fined. As someone who takes insulin I was horrified to hear this verdict.*

Several people on insulin have been charged with this offence after a hypo at the wheel when the only 'drug' that they have used is insulin. It may seem very unfair but, for any victim of such an accident, it is no consolation that the person responsible was hypo rather than under the influence of illegal drugs or alcohol. These cases emphasise the importance of taking driving seriously.

The rules for driving are:

- Always check your blood glucose before driving;
- If it is low, eat or take a glucose drink before you drive;
- Always carry food in your car and have some immediately if you feel warning of a hypo;
- If you think you may be hypo, pull off the road immediately, stop the car, turn off the ignition and remove the key;
- Do not resume driving until you are sure your blood glucose is in the normal range.

> *I recently read a newspaper article that implied that people with diabetes who are breathalysed can produce a positive reading even though they have not been drinking alcohol. What does this mean?*

Diabetes has no effect on breathalyser tests for alcohol even if acetone is present on the breath. However, the Lion Alcolmeter, widely used by the police, does also measure ketones, though this does not interfere with the alcohol measurement. Anyone breathalysed by the police may also be told that they have ketones and that they should consult their own doctor. These ketones may be caused either by diabetes that is out of control or by a long period of fasting.

ALCOHOL

My boyfriend likes a pint of beer in the evening but has just been found to have diabetes. Does this mean he will have to give up drinking beer?

No. There is no reason why he should not continue to drink beer. However, beer contains sugar and he may notice a rise in blood glucose soon after drinking. Special 'diabetic' lager contains less carbohydrate but more alcohol, with the drawback of being more expensive and more potent. He should probably also avoid the 'strong' brews, which are often labelled as being low in carbohydrate, as these are higher in alcohol than the ordinary types of beer and lager. Low-alcohol and alcohol-free beers and lagers often contain a lot of sugar, so, if he decides to change to these, he should look for the ones also labelled as being low in sugar (see Table 2.4).

Overall, your boyfriend is probably better off drinking ordinary beer. He should be aware that any form of alcohol can cause hypos, which may be delayed until the following morning so it would be worth keeping a close eye on his blood glucose levels the next day.

My teenage son has had diabetes since the age of seven. He is now beginning to show interest in going out with his friends in the evening. What advice can you give him about alcohol?

Most people with diabetes drink alcohol and it is perfectly safe for them to do so. However, as your son is on insulin he must be aware of certain problems that alcohol can cause: in particular, alcohol can make hypos more serious. When someone goes hypo a number of hormones are produced that make the liver release glucose into the bloodstream. If that person has drunk some alcohol, even as little as two pints of beer or a double measure of spirits, the liver will not be able to release glucose and hypos will be more sudden and more severe.

In practice, alcoholic drinks that also contain carbohydrate tend to increase the glucose in the blood. So the overall effect of a particular alcoholic drink depends on the proportions of alcohol to carbohydrate. For instance, lemonade shandy (high carbohydrate, low alcohol) will have a different effect on blood glucose from vodka and diet tonic (low carbohydrate, high alcohol). Your son may notice that 'diabetic' lager is more likely than ordinary beer to cause a hypo because it contains less carbohydrate but more alcohol.

If your son has been drinking in the evening, his blood glucose may drop in the early hours of the morning. To counteract this it would be sensible for him to eat a sandwich or cereal and milk to provide extra carbohydrate before going to bed. There is also evidence that after a night drinking alcohol, the risk of hypo is greatest the following morning and he should reduce his dose of pre-breakfast insulin and check his blood glucose level.

> *I like to go out with my friends a couple of nights a week and I usually end up drinking quite a bit. I've been told about alcohol and hypos but I've noticed that depending on what I drink, but especially when I'm drinking beer, my blood sugars can go really high before I get to bed. Is there anything I can do to stop this happening?*

Beer contains both sugar and alcohol. In general, the sugar causes an initial rise in the blood glucose level but the alcohol can lead to a hypo later. People respond differently to drinking alcohol and you need to monitor its effect on you as an individual. You need to check your blood glucose before and after drinking alcohol to help you work out your own requirements. If you find that your blood glucose rises consistently after beer, you may want to try to limit this rise.

You need to be cautious when experimenting with insulin doses. We suggest that you do nothing for the first couple of drinks but if you have more than this, you could try taking 1 unit of fast-acting insulin for every 20 g of carbohydrate (1 pint of beer = 13 g). You should remember the increased risk of a hypo later, which is greatest the following morning. To prevent this, you should try reducing your fast-acting insulin with breakfast or eat extra carbohydrate. This may be even more important if you have been very physically active.

I am 18 and go out a lot with my friends. I am careful never to drink and drive but, when it is not my turn to drive, I do drink quite a lot. I am careful not to miss any meals and I am not increasing my insulin as I used to when I first started drinking, but I have had quite a few bad hypos recently. Why should this happen?

This is because alcohol blocks the release of glucose from the liver (see the previous question). If your blood glucose is dropping because it is a while since you have eaten or because you have been out and active longer than usual, your body will not be able to come to the rescue as normal. Ideally it would be better if you could try not to have more than three or four units of alcohol in any one session. One unit of alcohol is equivalent to the following:

- half a pint of beer or lager or cider;
- one glass of wine;
- one single pub measure of spirits;
- one measure of sherry or aperitif.

If you are going to have more than three or four units in one session, make sure that you have your usual meal before you go out, have a snack while out and, very importantly, have a sandwich before you go to bed. Following this plan will help prevent you having hypos. There is also the risk of delayed hypos the morning after drinking and you may have to reduce your pre-breakfast insulin dose.

I have read that I can drink 'in moderation', but what does that really mean?

There are recommended safe drinking limits whether or not you have diabetes. The maximum healthy weekly limits are 21 units for men and 14 units for women. This is up to 3–4 units for men and 2–3 units for women each day. The answer to the previous question gives some examples of units of alcohol. If you use mixers, try to have the low-calorie varieties such as Slimline tonic or soda water, or diet lemonade. Remember that alcohol is high in calories, so if you are trying to lose weight you need to watch the amount you drink. Alcohol can also make hypos more serious so always make sure you have something to eat if you are going to have more than a couple of drinks. It may be safer to have a snack at bedtime to avoid this.

DRUGS

My son was told that people with diabetes should not use Betnovate cream because it contains steroids. Is this true and why?

It is best to avoid using powerful steroid creams such as Betnovate® unless there is a serious skin condition. Very often a weak steroid preparation or some bland ointment is just as effective in clearing up mild patches of eczema and other rashes. Unfortunately, too often the very strong steroids are used first, instead of as a last resort. These strong steroids can be absorbed into the body through the skin and lead to a number of unwanted side effects. This applies to all people with skin problems and not just people with diabetes. One of the side effects of steroids is a rise in the blood glucose level. Thus, someone without diabetes may develop it while taking steroids and a person treated with diet only may need to go onto tablets or insulin.

If there are good medical reasons for your son to take steroids, in whatever form, he should test his blood for signs of poor control and increase his insulin if necessary.

Can you tell me if any vaccinations including BCG are dangerous for people with diabetes?

There is no reason why a child should not have full immunisation against the usual childhood diseases. Sometimes inoculation is followed by a mild flu-like illness, which may lead to a slight upset of diabetes control. In some areas school children are given BCG as a protection against tuberculosis.

Children should also have the normal immunisation procedures if they travel to exotic places (see the section *Holidays and travel* earlier in this chapter).

My partner suffers from bad indigestion. She is afraid to take indigestion tablets in case they upset her diabetes. Can you advise her what to do?

Indigestion tablets and medicines do not upset diabetes.

Is it safe to take water tablets with diabetes?

Water tablets (diuretics) are given to people who are retaining too much fluid in the body. This fluid retention may happen in heart failure and cause swelling of the ankles or shortness of breath. Diuretics are usually very effective but, as a side effect, they may cause a slight increase in the blood glucose. This is especially true of the milder diuretics from the thiazide group such as bendroflumethiazide. The increase in glucose is only slight and although someone with diabetes controlled by diet alone may need to take tablets, people already on insulin should not notice any effect. The thiazide group of tablets is also used in the treatment of raised blood pressure.

Is there any special cough mixture for people with diabetes?

There are various sugar-free cough mixtures that can be bought from your chemist. However, there is only a tiny bit of sugar in a dose of ordinary cough mixture and this amount will not have any appreciable effect on the level of blood glucose.

I have been on insulin for diabetes for seven years. I was recently found to have raised blood pressure and was given tablets, called beta-blockers, by my doctor. Since then I have had a bad hypo in which I collapsed without the normal warning signs of sweating, shaking, etc. Could the blood pressure tablets have caused this severe hypo?

Beta-blockers are widely used for the treatment of high blood pressure and certain heart conditions. They have an 'anti-adrenaline' effect, which theoretically could damp down the normal 'adrenaline' response to a hypo (see the section *Hypos* in Chapter 3). However, research has shown that beta-blockers do not reduce the adrenaline warning of a hypo. Some beta-blockers have been designed to have their effect mainly on the heart without blocking the general adrenaline reaction. These selective beta-blockers, such as atenolol or bisoprolol, are theoretically safer for people taking insulin.

Please could you give me a list of tablets or medicines that may interfere with my diabetes?

The important medicines that affect diabetes have already been discussed in this section. There are no medicines that must never be used but the following might increase the blood glucose and upset your control:

- steroids (e.g. prednisolone, Betnovate® ointment, Becotide® inhaler) may cause a rise in blood glucose level but inhalers or ointment will only have this effect if taken in large doses;

- thiazide diuretics (e.g. bendroflumethiazide);

- the contraceptive pill;

- hormone replacement therapy;

- certain bronchodilators (e.g. Ventolin®) might have a slight effect of raising the blood glucose;

- growth hormone treatment.

SMOKING

I am a 16-year-old on insulin. I would like to know whether smoking low tar cigarettes could interfere with my diabetes. Would it cause any restriction in my diet?

Smoking is unhealthy because it may cause several cancers, and hardening of the arteries – affecting the heart, brain and legs. The best advice to all people, including teenagers, is not to smoke. Smoking will not directly affect your diabetes except, perhaps, by reducing your appetite (but see answer below).

When my doctor saw me for a review of my diabetes, he told me to stop smoking. Could you tell me if there is a particular health hazard associated with smoking and diabetes? The problem is made worse for me by the fact that I need to lose weight and, if I stop smoking, I will do just the opposite.

Smoking is a danger, both to the lungs and because of the risk of increased arterial disease, which affects anyone who smokes. Someone with long-standing diabetes is at risk of problems with poor blood circulation, and it is unwise to increase this risk by continuing to smoke.

There is a lot of support available now for people who want to give up smoking, and your GP or practice nurse should be able to offer you advice on whom to contact. They may run a group or clinic to help you quit. Some people are helped by nicotine gum or patches and we deal with these in a later question in this section.

Since my partner, who has had diabetes for 23 years, has stopped smoking, he has had high blood glucose tests. Why is this?

Your partner should be congratulated for giving up smoking. Most people who give up smoking put on weight, on average 4 kg (9 lb). This is because cigarettes suppress the appetite and make the body operate less efficiently, thus burning up more fuel (food). If he is eating more, his blood glucose levels will rise and he will need to increase his insulin to deal with this.

My doctor has strongly advised me to give up smoking and suggested that I try nicotine patches. I was surprised to find that the information leaflet enclosed with the patches advised people with diabetes not to use the patches. Is this true?

It sounds as though the manufacturer is being overcautious. The main reason for giving up smoking is to reduce the damage that it does to the blood supply to the heart, brain and legs. With each cigarette smoked, the nicotine inhaled narrows the small blood vessels. This narrowing eventually becomes permanent, which explains why smoking increases the risk of heart attacks, strokes and gangrene. Nicotine patches have been shown to be a most effective way of helping people to stop smoking.

Nicotine has the same effect on the blood vessels whether from patches or from cigarettes. However, patches are no worse than cigarettes and, if they help you to give up smoking, the overall benefit will be enormous, especially with regard to your circulation. Don't be afraid to try nicotine patches in the recommended dose. The same advice applies to nicotine chewing gum and the newer nicotine inhaler.

PRESCRIPTION CHARGES
AND SOCIAL SECURITY BENEFITS

*I believe that people with diabetes are entitled to free
prescriptions. Please could you tell me how to apply?*

One of the few advantages of having diabetes is exemption from
payment on all prescription charges – even for treatment uncon-
nected with the diabetes itself. People treated on diet alone are not
exempt from prescription charges.

You must obtain a form, called *NHS prescriptions – how to get them
free*, from your GP. The completed form should be signed by your doctor who will send it to the Primary Care Trust (PCT). You will then
receive an exemption certificate. Please remember to carry this certificate wherever you are likely to need a prescription, for example
travelling in the UK. The certificate lasts for five years, and you will
then need to renew it.

*What Social Security benefits am I entitled to now that I have
diabetes?*

There are no special benefits given automatically to people with
diabetes. You may claim Disability Living Allowance if you have
a child with diabetes who is under the age of 12, and it may be possible to obtain this allowance for a child up to the age of 16 if you can
prove that the child needs extra supervision and care. Diabetes UK
Careline can provide you with information to help you complete the
necessary forms.

For more information about benefits, we suggest that you contact
either Diabetes UK Careline, the Disability Alliance (addresses in
Appendix 2), or the Benefits Agency. This organisation deals with
Social Security benefits on behalf of the Department for Work and
Pensions, and you can make enquiries either at its offices or by
phone. You will find the addresses and telephone numbers (there are

several freephone enquiry lines) in your local phone book under 'Benefits Agency'. From the homepage of the website: www.direct.gov.uk you can go straight to 'money, tax and benefits'.

> *Since developing diabetes I have found that my food bills have risen alarmingly. Are there any special allowances that I can claim to offset the very high cost of the food?*

Most people with diabetes are not entitled to any special allowance and, indeed, there is no real need for them to eat different food from others. Special diabetic products are not necessary. Now that people are encouraged to eat food that is high rather than low in carbohydrate, they do not have to fall back on expensive protein as a source of calories. There is a question in the *Diet* section of Chapter 2 offering suggestions on keeping down the cost of food (see p. 28).

> *My mother has had diabetes for 12 years and is subject to crashing hypos for no reason. She needs someone to be with her all the time. Would we be eligible for an Attendance Allowance as she needs watching 24 hours a day?*

If you have to provide a continuous watch over your mother, you can apply for an Attendance Allowance. Before admitting defeat, however, it would be better to try every means of preventing the hypos. Presumably your mother is having insulin, though you do not mention the dose or type of insulin. It would be worth checking with the local diabetes service if anything could be done to reduce the frequency of hypos. Changing to more frequent but smaller doses of insulin might solve the problem. You may have to spend time and energy getting to grips with your mother's diabetes. It would do more for her self-confidence to abolish the hypos than to get an Attendance Allowance.

Sometimes people who are developing Alzheimer's disease are at risk of hypos because they forget to eat at the correct time. We know someone who has overcome this problem by wearing a watch with a timer, which can be set to ring an alarm at mealtimes. One such device is called a MedicAlarm – see Appendix 2.

MISCELLANEOUS

Is there any objection to my donating blood? I am on two injections of soluble insulin a day and my general health is fine.

It is hard to understand why a fit person with diabetes should not be a blood donor. However, the blood transfusion authorities do not accept blood from people on insulin. They suggest that the antibodies to insulin found in all people having injections may in some way harm the recipient of the blood.

Is it true that someone with diabetes should not use an electric blanket?

It is perfectly safe for you to use an electric blanket, although most underblankets should be used only to warm up the bed in advance. The manufacturers usually recommend that underblankets should be switched off before you get into bed. However, there are now underblankets that can be left on all night on a very low heat and these would be safe to use, provided that you follow the manufacturer's instructions. Overblankets can be left on all night, but again you should always check the manufacturer's instructions.

Hot-water bottles are rather more dangerous as their temperature is not controlled. People with a slight degree of nerve damage can fail to realise that a bottle full of very hot water may be burning the skin of their feet. This is a recognised cause of foot ulcers. It is better to be safe than sorry and avoid the comfort of a hot-water bottle. Bedsocks are a possible alternative for cold feet, or you could try one of the small electric heating pads now on the market. Again you need to be careful how you use these and follow the manufacturer's instructions – not all of them are suitable for use in bed.

My 10-year-old daughter has had diabetes for three months. She has started to lose a lot of hair and now has a bald patch. Is this connected with her diabetes?

Yes, it could be. There are three ways in which diabetes and hair loss may be connected.

- If your daughter was very ill with ketoacidosis at the time of her diagnosis, this could lead to a heavy loss of hair. In this case, her hair will regrow over the next few months.

- Alopecia areata is a skin condition which is slightly more common in people with diabetes. This is the likely diagnosis if your daughter has a well-defined bald patch with the rest of her hair remaining a normal thickness. If the patch is on the top of her head, there is a chance that her hair will regrow over the next six months. There is no way of encouraging growth and steroid ointments may cause permanent skin changes and make matters worse.

- Lack of thyroid hormones may occur with diabetes. If this is the cause of your daughter's hair loss, you will notice other symptoms such as mental slowing, weight increase and an inability to keep warm. All these symptoms can be corrected by taking thyroid tablets. A simple blood test will identify the condition.

Shortage of body iron may also cause hair loss although this is not connected with diabetes.

I recently enquired about having electrolysis treatment for excess hair. I was told that, as I had diabetes, I would need a letter from my doctor stating that my diabetes did not encourage hair growth. Could I use wax hair removers instead?

There is no objection to your having electrolysis. Diabetes does not cause excessive hair growth. It sounds as though the firm doing the electrolysis is being overcautious.

People with diabetes can use the same methods of hair removal as those without diabetes – no special precautions are needed.

Is it safe for people with diabetes to use sunbeds and saunas?

It is as safe as for those without diabetes: exposure to ultraviolet radiation is known to increase the risk of skin cancer. If you do use one, make sure that you can recognise the signs of a hypo when you are hot and sweaty. Keep some means of treating a hypo with you – not with your clothes in the changing room.

I have diabetes and would dearly love to have my ears pierced but, when I asked my doctor about this, he said there was a chance that my ears would swell. Please could you advise me if there is a great risk of this happening?

Anyone who has their ears pierced runs a small risk of infection until the wound heals completely. The risk in a person with well controlled diabetes is no higher than normal. If your ears do become red, swollen and painful, you may need an antibiotic.

Is there any connection between vertigo and diabetes?

Vertigo, in the strict medical sense, describes the sensation when the world seems to be spinning round. It is usually due to disease of the inner ear or of the part of the brain that controls balance. This is not connected with diabetes in any way. However, simple dizzy spells are a common problem with many possible causes, which may be difficult to diagnose. If dizziness occurs when you move from sitting down to standing, it may be the result of a sudden fall in blood pressure. This can sometimes be due to a loss of reflexes as a result of diabetic neuropathy (see Chapter 9: **Long-term complications** for more information about neuropathy). There are no other connections between diabetes and vertigo.

My partner's grandmother is 84 and has diabetes. Although she is fiercely independent, she cannot look after herself properly and will have to go into a residential home. Can you let me know of any homes that cater especially for people with diabetes?

Because diabetes is becoming increasingly common in the elderly, the staff in most residential homes are experienced in looking after people with diabetes. They will probably be happy to do blood tests, ensure that her diet is satisfactory and arrange for her to be given insulin injections if she is unable to do this herself.

My wife, who developed diabetes a few weeks ago, is about to return to work. I feel that she should wear some sort of identity disc or bracelet showing that she has diabetes but she is reluctant to wear anything too eye-catching. Have you any suggestions?

It is very important that all people with diabetes, especially those on insulin, should wear some form of identification. Accidents do happen and it may be vital for any medical emergency team to know that your wife has diabetes.

Medic-Alert provides stainless steel bracelets or necklets which are functional if not very beautiful. They can also be obtained in silver, gold plate, and 9-carat gold. Medic-Alert's address is in Appendix 2.

SOS/Talisman (address is in Appendix 2) produces a medallion which can be unscrewed to reveal identification and medical details. These can be bought in most jewellers and come in a wide range of styles and prices, including some in 9-carat gold. Other products are always coming onto the market, and *Balance*, the magazine produced by Diabetes UK, usually carries advertisements.

Could you tell me what ointment to use for skin irritation?

The most common cause of skin irritation in people with diabetes is itching around the genital region (pruritus vulvae). The most important treatment is to eliminate glucose from the urine by controlling diabetes. However, the itching can be relieved temporarily by cream containing a fungicide (e.g. nystatin).

> *I have recently been given a foot spa and was surprised to see a caution on the side of the box that it is not suitable for people with diabetes. Is this true?*

If you have neuropathy (nerve damage), you should check with your diabetes team before using the spa. If you don't have neuropathy, make sure that you check the temperature of the water carefully and don't soak your feet for too long as this will make the skin soggy, easily damaged and prone to infection.

6 | Sex, contraception and HRT

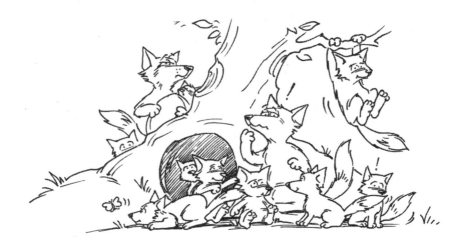

These days there is a more relaxed attitude to discussing subjects such as sex and contraception, but many people still find it difficult to ask questions about these topics. Generally, people with diabetes are no different from those without diabetes in any aspect of sexuality, fertility, infertility and contraception. However, there are some problems, such as the increased risk of impotence (sometimes known as erectile dysfunction) in men who have had diabetes for many years. This is often caused by neuropathy (nerve damage) or poor blood supply. Nowadays there are a variety of treatments available and if you are concerned about erectile dysfunction you should speak to your doctor. There have been very few studies of the effect of diabetes on sexual function in women but there is some evidence to suggest that women who have had diabetes for many years may have more difficulty achieving orgasm.

Various contraceptive devices have at times been said to be less effective in women with diabetes – the evidence for this is poor and women with diabetes should choose their contraception depending on their personal preferences. Some oral contraceptive pills may be more suitable than others but your doctor will be able to advise you. Oral contraceptives do not increase the risk of developing diabetes.

IMPOTENCE

I am a middle-aged man with diabetes. I have been told that diabetes could affect my sex life. Is this correct?

Most people with diabetes, both male and female, lead a completely normal and full sex life. It is true that problems may occur but many of these have nothing to do with diabetes. If your blood glucose levels are consistently high, this could affect your sex life. Some men have either nerve damage or arterial disease causing loss of sexual potency (erectile dysfunction), which can be directly attributed to diabetes.

Is it normal for people with diabetes to suddenly find themselves totally uninterested in sexual intercourse? My husband is really upset about my lack of desire!

The feeling that you describe is more common in women than men, but is no more likely in women with diabetes. Anything which makes you tired can lead to loss of interest in sex and poorly controlled diabetes can certainly affect your energy levels. In these circumstances loss of interest in sex is one of casualties of the high blood glucose.

I have had erratic blood glucose levels recently. Would low blood glucose affect my ability to achieve or maintain an erection and more importantly, my ability to ejaculate?

Not unless the blood glucose is very low (less than 4 mmol/L), in which case many aspects of brain and nerve function are affected and this could reduce both your potency and ability to ejaculate. These will return to normal when your blood glucose is stable.

Am I likely to become impotent? I have had diabetes for five years.

There is no doubt that many men with diabetes worry about the possibility of developing erectile dysfunction (impotence) in the future. Our advice is to try to keep your diabetes under good control and this will reduce the risk of future complications. If you are unlucky enough to develop erectile difficulties, there are now a number of treatments available to help. Your doctor will be able to advise you and if necessary refer you to a specialist clinic.

My husband, who is middle-aged with Type 1 diabetes, has been impotent for the past two years. Please will you explain his condition as I am afraid that my teenage son, who also has diabetes, may worry that he is at risk of becoming impotent.

Erectile dysfunction (impotence) worries many people and occurs in men with and without diabetes. It appears that one in five men with diabetes may develop this problem at some stage in their lives, though the condition may be reversible. Most men with erectile difficulties do not have diabetes and a number of other factors such as anxiety, depression, overwork, tiredness, stress, alcohol excess and grief can cause this problem. Any man may find that he is temporarily impotent and fear of failure can make things worse. Overwork or worry can lead to lack of interest in sex and erectile dysfunction. Excess alcohol, while not causing lack of interest in sex, may lead to impotence.

Some men with diabetes do develop erectile difficulties, as a result of problems with the blood supply or the nerve supply to the penis. This usually develops slowly and in younger people it can often be prevented by strict blood glucose control. Treatments such as Viagra® are now available and can be prescribed by your doctor. In older people the condition is more difficult to treat successfully, partly because there may be other medical factors in addition to diabetes. You should discuss the matter further with your own doctor.

Recently, I have had trouble keeping an erection – has this anything to do with my diabetes? I also had a vasectomy a few years ago.

This is difficult to answer without knowing more about you and your medical history. Vasectomy may lead to impotence for psychological reasons but is unlikely to have caused any damage which might affect erections. Failure to maintain an adequate erection may be an early sign of diabetic neuropathy and you might need blood tests to rule out other medical causes. However, it is often a symptom of overwork or simply the ageing process.

I suffered a stroke affecting the right side of my body 12 months ago at the age of 40 and now suffer from partial impotence. The onset seemed to coincide not with the stroke but with taking anticoagulants. Are these known to cause impotence? I have also heard that blood pressure tablets can cause impotence and I have been taking these for three months. Could this be a factor?

A severe stroke can sometimes lead to impotence. A stroke is often due to narrowing of the arteries inside the head and the arteries elsewhere may also be narrowed. If those supplying blood to the penis are affected, this could contribute to your erectile dysfunction. You are also quite right about the drugs. Some blood pressure lowering drugs may cause impotence and can interfere with ejaculation. It would be unwise to stop taking the drugs since this would lead to loss of control of your blood pressure and the risk of a further stroke. However, there is individual variation in the way people respond to different tablets and you could ask your doctor if there are any alternative blood pressure tablets you could try. Anticoagulant tablets are not known to cause impotence.

I have been impotent for months. Is there some drug or hormone that will help me?

It is rare for a hormonal abnormality to cause impotence although it is normal practice to check the hormone levels by a blood test in any man with erectile dysfunction. If your impotence is caused by a hormonal deficiency, treatment with the replacement hormone (testosterone) may cure the problem. It is essential to get a correct diagnosis in order to ensure appropriate therapy. Many cases of impotence are due to psychological causes and often respond to appropriate advice or to drug treatment. Injecting a drug called Caverject® directly into the penis can sometimes be helpful. It leads to an immediate erection and the result is often good enough to make this an acceptable form of therapy.

Viagra® is the first oral treatment for impotence to be licensed in the UK. It works by helping to relax the blood vessels in the penis, allowing more blood to flow into the penis causing an erection and will only be effective if the man is sexually stimulated. It is available on the NHS, but officially the amount is limited to four tablets a month. It is important to use the full strength (100 mg) as lower amounts are much less likely to work. Viagra does have some strange side effects which you should ask about when it is prescribed.

I have heard about Weekend Viagra. Could you tell me more?

One of the drawbacks with Viagra® is that it only has its effect from one to three hours after taking the tablet. This may take much of the spontaneity out of sex. A newer tablet called Cialis® starts to have effect in 30 minutes and lasts for 36 hours – as the manufacturer claims 'for the best part of a weekend'. Levitra® is another drug similar to Viagra which should be taken 25–60 minutes before you want to have sex.

I have heard that Viagra may be dangerous and cause heart attacks. Is this true?

Apart from the obvious answer about sex and heart attacks, Viagra and the other drugs in the same group do not normally have a bad effect on the heart – in fact Viagra was first developed as a drug to help heart disease. There is one very important occasion when Viagra may be dangerous for people with angina. If they are taking any form of nitrate, including a nitrate (GTN) spray, they should not take Viagra as this may cause sudden collapse. Commonly used nitrates are Suscard®, isosorbide and Imdur®. If you think you may be taking a nitrate for angina, please check with your doctor before taking Viagra. Since nitrates prevent angina, it is not really safe to stop taking them in order to be able to have sex stimulated by Viagra.

I have used Viagra for three years for impotence. At first it worked very well but the effect now seems to be wearing off. Is there anything else I can try?

There is another drug on the market, which is designed to help men achieve an erection. It is called apomorphine (or Uprima®), and should be placed under the tongue about 20 minutes before you want to have sex. Apomorphine has about the same success rate as Viagra, but may help some men who do not respond to Viagra. Apomorphine seems to be a safe drug, but you should avoid it if you have severe heart problems or if your blood pressure is low.

Is there any other treatment for impotence apart from Viagra?

Depending on the cause, there are several effective forms of therapy. Counselling by a therapist trained in this subject can be helpful, particularly in cases where the stresses and conflicts of life are the root cause. Testosterone should help men with a deficiency of this hormone. Vacuum therapy, with a device that looks like a rigid condom, can be very successful but does require a sense of humour in both partners. Injections of papaverine or alprostadil (Caverject®) into the penis, and penile implants (which require an operation) are also effective. Choosing the best option for you as a couple requires a considerable amount of thought and discussion, both with your partner and your doctor. Many diabetes departments hold special clinics for treatment of impotence.

After sexual intercourse I recently suffered quite a bad hypo. Is this likely to happen again and if so, what can be done to prevent it?

Like any physical activity, sex can lower the blood glucose and lead to hypoglycaemia. When this happens, and it is not at all uncommon, you need to deal with the hypo in the usual way using fruit juice or Lucozade® (see section *Hypos* in Chapter 3). You may find it useful to keep some quick-acting carbohydrate close at hand.

CONTRACEPTION AND VASECTOMY

I have diabetes and want to start on the Pill. Are there any extra risks that women with diabetes run in using it?

The oral contraceptive pill is as effective for women with diabetes as for those without diabetes. It is now well known that the Pill carries a small risk of venous thrombosis, sometimes called DVT or deep vein thrombosis (where a vein becomes blocked by a blood clot) and pulmonary embolus (where the blood clot moves to the lung). To keep these risks to a minimum, you should take the smallest possible dose of oestrogen and your doctor will be able to advise you about the most suitable preparation. Some women are at higher risk and this includes those with a previous history of DVT or pulmonary embolus, smokers over the age of 35 years and those at high risk of stroke or heart attack. This last group includes women with a family history of heart disease or stroke at an early age and those with a high cholesterol or high blood pressure.

In general there is no reason why women with diabetes should not take the Pill, but if you have complications of diabetes such as high blood pressure, high cholesterol or kidney disease you may be at greater risk and you should consider an alternative method of contraception. The risk involved in pregnancy itself is greater than that of the Pill, so if you decide that the Pill is not for you it is important that you choose an effective alternative. Women with uncomplicated diabetes may certainly use the Pill and there are no additional risks.

When women with diabetes start using the Pill there is sometimes a slight deterioration of control. This is rarely a problem and is usually easily dealt with by a small increase in treatment, which in those taking insulin may mean a small increase in the dose. It is a simple matter to monitor the blood and make appropriate adjustments.

My doctor prescribed the Pill for me but on the packet it states that it is unsuitable for people with diabetes. As my doctor knows that I have diabetes is it safe enough for me?

There used to be some confusion about whether the Pill was suitable for women with diabetes but there is now general agreement that as long as there are no diabetes complications, they may use the Pill for contraceptive purposes without any increased risks compared with those who do not have diabetes. If you do have any diabetes-related complications you should speak to your doctor.

I want to try the progesterone-only contraceptive pill. Is it suitable for women with diabetes?

Yes, although this type of Pill has a higher failure rate than the combined pill so it has become less popular.

I have just started the menopause and wondered if I have to wait two years after my last period before doing away with contraception.

Although periods may become irregular and infrequent at the start of the menopause, it is still possible to be fertile, and this advice is a precaution against unwanted pregnancy. It applies equally to women with or without diabetes.

I have diabetes and I am marrying a man with diabetes in eight weeks' time. Please could you advise me on how to stop becoming pregnant?

We are not quite clear whether you wish to be sterilised and never have children or whether you are seeking contraceptive advice. If you and your fiancé have decided that you do not want to have the anxiety of your children inheriting diabetes and have made a clear decision not to have children, you have the option of your fiancé having a vasectomy or being sterilised yourself.

These are very fundamental decisions and will require careful thought because they are probably best considered as irreversible procedures. If you are quite certain about not having children, we would advise you both to discuss this with your GP and seek referral either to a surgeon for vasectomy for your fiancé or to a gynaecologist for sterilisation. Whichever you decide, you must both attend since no surgeon will undertake this procedure without being convinced that you have thought about it carefully and have come to a clear, informed decision.

If our interpretation of your question has not been right and you are simply looking for contraceptive advice, then the best source of this is either your GP or local family planning clinic. All the usual forms of contraceptives are suitable for women with diabetes, so it is just a question of discovering which best suits you and your partner.

Can you please give me any information regarding vasectomy and any side effects it may have for men with diabetes?

Vasectomy is a relatively minor surgical procedure, which involves cutting and tying off the vas deferens – the tube that carries sperm from the testes to the penis. Vasectomy may be carried out under either local or general anaesthetic usually as a day case. It would be simpler to have it under local anaesthetic as this will not disturb the balance of your diabetes. The main side effect of the operation is discomfort, which may last for a few days although infections and other complications do rarely occur.

There are a few medical reasons for avoiding this operation but they apply equally to men without diabetes as they do to men with diabetes and your doctor will be able to discuss these with you.

I have been warned that IUDs are more unreliable in women with diabetes. Is this really true?

IUDs (intrauterine contraceptive devices) are generally regarded as slightly less reliable contraceptives than the Pill, and there has been one report suggesting they may be even less reliable when used by women with diabetes. No other studies have backed up this observation. There has also been a report suggesting that women with diabetes may be slightly more susceptible to pelvic infections when using an IUD. On balance, we believe that IUDs should be considered effective and useful in women with diabetes.

THRUSH

I keep getting recurrence of vaginal thrush and my doctor says that, as I have diabetes, there is nothing that I can do about this – is this correct?

Thrush is due to an infection with a yeast (*Candida*) that thrives in the presence of a lot of glucose. If your diabetes is badly controlled and you are passing a lot of glucose in your urine, you will be very susceptible to vaginal thrush and, however much ointment and cream you use, it is likely to recur. The best treatment is to control your diabetes so well that there is no glucose in your urine, but if the thrush persists, you will need antifungal treatment from your doctor. If you keep your urine free from glucose, you should stay free from further thrush infections.

I suffer with thrush. My diabetes has been well controlled for ten years now. I do regular blood tests and most of them are less than 10 mmol/L and, whenever I check a urine test, it is always negative. I have been taking the oral contraceptive pill for three years and I understand that both diabetes and the Pill can lead to thrush. Can you advise me what to do?

Since your diabetes is well controlled and your urine consistently free from glucose, diabetes can probably be ruled out as a cause of the thrush. It sounds as if you are either being reinfected by your partner or alternatively it is an uncommon side effect of the Pill, and you should discuss a change of contraception with your doctor.

HORMONE REPLACEMENT THERAPY (HRT)

Can you tell me if hormone replacement therapy for the menopause is suitable for women with diabetes?

Hormone replacement therapy (HRT) for the menopause consists of small doses of oestrogen and progesterone given to replace the hormones normally produced by the ovaries. Oestrogen levels in the blood begin to fall at the menopause and, if this happens rapidly, it can cause unpleasant symptoms, such as hot flushes. Replacement therapy is designed to allow a more gradual decline in the female hormones. There has been a lot of publicity about the adverse effects of HRT in the last few years and there is some evidence to suggest an increased risk of breast cancer, thrombosis and stroke. However, these risks have to be balanced against the benefits of HRT. The evidence shows that for every 1000 women taking combined oestrogen and progestogen replacement therapy for five years, there will be:

- six extra cases of breast cancer;
- nine extra cases of thrombosis (blood clots) in the legs or in the lungs;
- two extra cases of of stroke.

Women with diabetes already have an increased risk of stroke and heart attack and HRT may increase this. The current advice is that women with severe menopausal symptoms benefit from short-term HRT but for those without symptoms the risks outweigh the benefits. In the past, HRT has been recommended for prevention of osteoporosis but since it may be responsible for the unwanted side effects listed above, some experts recommend that other preventative treatments are used in preference to HRT.

These are not easy decisions but doctors are now cautious about recommending HRT routinely to all women. As the risks of stroke are greater for women with diabetes, we would advise that HRT is only used by women with severe menopausal symptoms, and for as short a period as possible.

I want to try and avoid osteoporosis by taking HRT. As I have diabetes, is this sensible?

HRT is the most effective treatment for the prevention of osteo- porosis but because of the problems mentioned in the previous question, some doctors are cautious about recommending it as a first choice. The decision depends on your individual risk of developing osteoporosis. If you have a high risk, you may choose to take HRT and accept the small chance of unwanted complications; if your risk is low, you may prefer to try an alternative, which may be less effec- tive but lessen your chances of complications. Please speak to your doctor about this. You should, of course, take general measures such as ensuring adequate calcium in your diet and taking regular weight-bearing exercise.

Are the patch forms of HRT as suitable for women with diabetes as the tablets?

There is no known difference between tablets and patches; all the answers to the questions above apply equally to patches.

TERMINATION OF PREGNANCY

I have become pregnant and really don't want a baby at the moment. Is diabetes grounds for termination of pregnancy?

No, not unless your doctor considers that the pregnancy would be detrimental to your health, which may sometimes be the case if you have complications of diabetes. If you do not have any complica- tions the reasons for termination of pregnancy apply equally to women with and without diabetes.

I am going into hospital for an abortion. I am worried that the doctors might not do it as I have diabetes. Should I have told someone?

There is no added hazard for women with diabetes who undergo termination of pregnancy, and care of the diabetes during this operation does not raise any special difficulties. It is still important to tell your gynaecologist that you have diabetes so that good control can be maintained during this time.

FERTILITY

I have recently got married and my wife and I are keen to start a family. Are people with diabetes more likely to be infertile?

There is nothing to suggest that men with diabetes are any less fertile than men who do not have diabetes and in general this is also true for women. However, women with consistently high blood glucose readings may find it more difficult to conceive. This may be a good thing as there is sound evidence to show that the outcome of pregnancy is much worse in women who conceive when their control is poor.

I have been trying for a baby for years and we have now decided to go for fertility counselling and possible treatment. Can people with diabetes expect the same treatment for infertility as people without?

Yes. As mentioned in the previous question, diabetes is rarely the cause of infertility. If control is anything other than excellent, improving control, aiming for an HbA_{1c} of less than 7.5% should be the first goal. Referral to a fertility expert is the next step but good control would be necessary before treatment could be started.

7 | Pregnancy

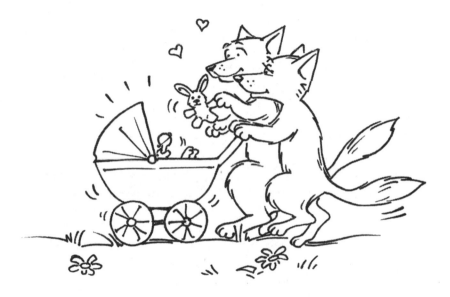

Pregnancy was the first condition associated with diabetes where it was proved that poor blood glucose control led to complications for both mother and child and that these complications could be avoided by strict blood glucose control. The outcome for pregnant women with diabetes, and for their babies, is directly related to how well they control their blood glucose throughout the pregnancy. If control is good from the moment of conception to delivery, the risks to mother and baby can be little greater than in women without diabetes.

We now know that poor control at conception, when the egg is fertilised, can affect the way in which the egg divides and develops into the fetus (the stage at which all organs and limbs are present in minute form). This sometimes leads to congenital abnormalities such as spina bifida, hole in the heart and cleft palate. The risk of this happening can be reduced to a minimum, and possibly eliminated, by ensuring a normal HbA_{1c} before becoming pregnant. The evidence suggests that the higher the HbA_{1c} at conception, the higher the risk of an abnormality in the baby.

Some of these problems may be detected by ultrasound scan early in pregnancy, and termination may be considered if a major defect is found. If the scan shows a normal fetus, the outcome of the pregnancy will still be affected by the mother's blood glucose control during the rest of her pregnancy. Poor control tends to lead to big babies and this can be a problem for both mother and baby at the time of delivery. Sadly, there is also a greater risk of stillbirth in babies of mothers with poor diabetes control but careful monitoring of the baby close to the time of delivery has greatly reduced this risk.

A recent audit of pregnancy in mothers with diabetes (CEMACH – Confidential Enquiry into Maternal and Child Health) has come up with some disappointing results. In the course of this national audit, information was collected from all 231 maternity units in England, Wales and Northern Ireland, and showed that despite increasing awareness of the need for good control, the results for pregnancies complicated by diabetes are still very unsatisfactory. Babies of mothers with diabetes are:

- five times more likely to be stillborn;
- twice as likely to have a congenital malformation;
- twice as likely to weigh more than 4 kg (9 lb).

This is true for both Type 1 and Type 2 diabetes. See the website: www.cemach.org.uk/publications for full details.

These figures are very disturbing and compare unfavourably with other countries, such as Australia. There is clearly need for improvement since we know that with careful attention to diabetes control and close monitoring of the baby, the outcome of the pregnancy can be much better.

Modern antenatal care is usually shared between the diabetes specialist and the obstetrician, preferably at a joint clinic. Admission to hospital is rarely necessary as long as the pregnancy progresses normally and control remains good, in which case the pregnancy should continue close to its natural term. Any antenatal complications will be treated in the same way as they would be in women without diabetes. Once spontaneous labour begins, the only difference from the normal process is the need to keep the mother's blood glucose normal to prevent hypoglycaemia in the baby after delivery. Although the aim should always be for a normal delivery, mothers with diabetes do have a higher chance of needing a Caesarean section, particularly if the baby is large or needs to be delivered early.

Most women are able to make the great effort required to keep tight control during pregnancy but it is very difficult to keep this up once they are faced with the demands of a new baby and the need to avoid hypoglycaemia.

A very comprehensive pregnancy magazine is available from Diabetes UK.

PREPREGNANCY

The man I am going to marry has Type 1 diabetes. Will any children we may have be at risk of developing diabetes?

If you do not have diabetes yourself and there is no diabetes in your family, the risk of your children developing diabetes in childhood or adolescence, if their father has diabetes, is probably about 1 in 20. Provided that you are both in good health it is certainly all right to have a family. If you and your fiancé both have Type 1 diabetes, there will be a greater risk of your children developing diabetes. Strangely enough, the risk of children developing diabetes is lower if the parent with diabetes is their mother, rather than their father.

There is a rare form of Type 2 diabetes in which there is a strong hereditary tendency. This is called maturity onset diabetes of the young, commonly known as MODY. Were you or your fiancé to have this, the risk of your children getting diabetes of this unusual kind would be rather high. It is often a relatively mild form of diabetes and runs true to type throughout the generations.

The study of inheritance of diabetes is a complicated subject and you would be well advised to discuss this further with your specialist or a professional genetic counsellor.

I am worried that, if I become pregnant while my husband's diabetes is uncontrolled, the child will suffer – am I right?

No. There is no known way in which poor control of your husband's diabetes can affect the development of your child.

I am 29 years old and have Type 1 diabetes. My partner and I plan to start a family but first I would like to complete a three-year degree course at university. By the time this course finishes I will be 32. Can you tell me if I shall then be too old to have a baby?

There is a trend nowadays for women to delay starting a family until they are well into their thirties. Thirty-two is not too old to have a child but if you have diabetes, there are some advantages in having children earlier rather than later. The main reason for this is that the longer you have had diabetes, the greater the risk of developing complications which may have a significant effect on the pregnancy.

Having said this, many women with diabetes have successful pregnancies in their thirties and even forties. It is difficult to give specific advice and the right person to talk to is your family doctor or diabetes specialist, who will know both you and your diabetes.

Why must I ensure that my diabetes control is perfect during pregnancy?

This is to ensure that you reduce the risks to yourself and your baby to an absolute minimum. If you are able to achieve this degree of control from before the time of conception through to the time of delivery, the risks to your baby are only slightly greater than those for babies born to women without diabetes. On the other hand, if your diabetes is poorly controlled, the risk to your baby increases dramatically.

I have diabetes and would like a pregnancy soon. I have heard that women who are planning a pregnancy should take tablets called folic acid. What are these for and should I take them?

Folic acid is a naturally occurring vitamin which is present in many foods. There is good evidence that if women take extra folic acid in the early stages of pregnancy, the risk of abnormalities of the nervous system, such as spina bifida, are reduced. For women without diabetes the recommended dose is 400 µg, but women with diabetes, who are at higher risk of having a baby with an abnormality, are advised to take the higher dose of 5 mg. Your doctor will be able to prescribe this for you.

PREGNANCY MANAGEMENT

When I had my first baby, I was in hospital for the last two months and had a Caesarean section at 36 weeks. My baby weighed 3.7 kg (8 lb 4 oz) even though she was four weeks early. During my most recent pregnancy I went into labour at 39 weeks and the baby weighed 3.2 kg (7 lb) – the only time I was in hospital was for the birth. Why was there such a big change in treatment?

The last 20 years have seen a dramatic change in our attitudes to the care of pregnant women with diabetes. Good blood glucose control is the most important goal and with home blood glucose monitoring the majority of women can achieve this without the need for admission to hospital. It sounds as if your control was better

during your second pregnancy than in your first. On the first occasion early delivery by Caesarean section was advised because the
baby had already grown to 3.7 kg by 36 weeks and the doctors were
worried that it would become even bigger if left to 38 or 39 weeks.
The baby was probably large because your blood glucose levels were
high, resulting in your baby becoming overweight and bloated.
During your most recent pregnancy, when your control was better,
the baby grew at a more normal rate, so that it was not necessary to
deliver you early and you were able to go into labour naturally.

*During my last labour I was given a drip and had an insulin
pump up all day. Why was this necessary?*

Strict blood glucose control during labour is very important to
ensure that you do not put your baby at risk from hypoglycaemia
in the first few hours of life. The drip and insulin pump is the most
effective way of ensuring this degree of control. In any labour there
is always a possibility that you may need an anaesthetic (e.g. for for-
ceps delivery or possible Caesarean section), and by using the insulin
pump your midwife can ensure that if an emergency arises you will
be immediately ready.

*During my pregnancy I found attending the antenatal clinic a
nuisance and I did not like to keep my diabetes too tightly
controlled because, if I did, I had a lot of hypos. I went into
labour naturally, but the delivery was difficult. I was told that
my baby's shoulders got stuck because he was so big. He had to
spend a long time in the Special Care Baby Unit because his
sugar was low. How do I avoid all this trouble in my next
pregnancy?*

We understand that attending the antenatal clinic frequently is
time-consuming and tedious, but the chances of a good pregnancy outcome are greatly increased by the careful monitoring you
receive at these clinic visits. Your baby's difficult delivery and long

admission to the Special Care Baby Unit might have been avoided if your diabetes had been better controlled and the growth of your baby had been monitored by scans.

Your baby was big because he had been exposed to a high glucose concentration throughout pregnancy and he had to produce a lot of insulin from his own pancreas to cope with this extra load of glucose from you. The extra glucose was converted to fat and this is what made him big. Immediately after birth he no longer had the glucose coming from you but still had too much insulin of his own, leading to hypoglycaemia. This complication can be avoided by keeping your blood glucose levels as normal as possible. Although we agree that this does increase your risk of hypos, it should be possible to find an insulin regimen which enables you to achieve good control without a lot of hypos and your diabetes team will be keen to help you with this.

Even with good blood glucose control, babies of mothers with diabetes are often bigger than average and this is detected by regular growth scans. Your doctors can then discuss the timing and method of delivery with you so that the difficulties you encountered in your last delivery can be avoided.

Is it all right for me to breastfeed my baby if my blood glucose is too high?

All women are encouraged to breastfeed as breast milk provides their babies with the best possible nutrition and protection against infection. There is no reason why diabetes should prevent you from breastfeeding and your baby will not be harmed in any way if your blood glucose is high. However, persistently high levels may cause you to become dehydrated, which can reduce milk production. For the best results with breastfeeding, keep up a high fluid intake and try to keep a check on your blood glucose to make sure it is neither very high nor very low. It is probably best to relax your diabetes control a little to make sure that you avoid hypos as it can be very difficult to cope with a new baby if you are constantly hypo.

Breastfeeding takes a lot of energy in terms of nutritional requirements, so try to make sure that you eat regular amounts of
carbohydrate. You will probably find that you need to increase your
calorie intake and take less than your usual pre-pregnancy dose of
insulin. Do not try to breastfeed while having a hypo: feed yourself
first, so that you can feed and look after your baby safely. Always seek
medical advice if you are in any doubt. If you find breastfeeding too
difficult, it is perfectly all right to bottle-feed.

*My diabetes was fairly easy to control during my pregnancy, but
since the birth of my baby it has been more difficult to control,
and I am needing much less insulin. I am breastfeeding – could
this have anything to do with it?*

During pregnancy the placenta produces large quantities of hormones which oppose the action of insulin, producing an insulin
resistant state. It is not unusual for women to need 2–3 times their
normal dose of insulin during the second half of pregnancy.
Surprisingly, the blood glucose levels actually become easier to control with fewer fluctuations, even though the overall insulin dose is
greater. After the birth the hormone levels fall immediately, which
means that your insulin dose returns to the pre-pregnancy level as
soon as the baby is born. In many women the dose needed in the first
few days is even lower than was required before pregnancy. When
you are breastfeeding, the dose usually drops even more and you
should be prepared to lower your dose of insulin as much as necessary to avoid hypos.

*I am married to a man who takes insulin to control his diabetes.
I have just become pregnant, so what special things do I need to
do during pregnancy to ensure that it goes smoothly and
without complications?*

You need take no special precautions other than those taken by
all pregnant women, as the fact that your husband has diabetes

does not put your pregnancy at any particular risk. It is only when the mother has diabetes that strict control and careful monitoring of blood glucose become essential.

I have been told that I must keep my blood glucose levels as low as possible during pregnancy. Please can you tell me what they should be?

Your blood glucose before meals should be 4–6 mmol/litre and you should aim to be no higher than 8 mmol/L two hours after meals. If you find that this is difficult to achieve without causing a lot of hypos you should discuss the problem with your diabetes team.

I am frightened of having hypoglycaemic attacks especially as I have been told to keep my blood glucose much lower during pregnancy. What should I do?

All people treated with insulin should be prepared for a hypo whether or not they are pregnant (see the section *Hypos* in Chapter 3) but the emphasis on tight control during pregnancy does increase the risk of hypo. Carry some form of rapidly absorbed glucose at all times – Dextro-Energy tablets are convenient. Some people prefer to carry small (125 mL) cans of Lucozade® or a cola drink (not diet cola.) Your partner should be shown how to use Glucogel® (formerly Hypostop Gel) and glucagon injections as these can reverse the hypo very rapidly. Make sure you always test your blood glucose before driving.

Will any hypoglycaemic attacks that I might have during pregnancy harm the baby?

There is no evidence to suggest that even a very low blood glucose in the mother can harm the baby.

COMPLICATIONS

My second son was born with multiple defects and later died. I have been on insulin for 14 years (since the age of 10). Are women with diabetes more likely to have an abnormal baby?

It is a terrible tragedy to lose a baby as a result of birth defects and we hope you can pick yourself up and approach your diabetes in a positive way. The secret to a successful pregnancy is excellent blood glucose control starting before conception and continuing throughout pregnancy. There is good scientific evidence to suggest that developmental defects are caused by poor control in the first few weeks of pregnancy and that the risk of this can be reduced by ensuring perfect control when the baby is conceived. This means aiming for an HbA_{1c} of less than 7.5%. The risk of multiple congenital defects is confined to the early stages of the pregnancy. This is hardly surprising because this is the stage when the various components of the baby's body are beginning to develop and when other illnesses such as German measles (rubella) can also affect development. However, this means that there is no time to improve control once you discover that you are pregnant and it is crucial to plan the pregnancy and make sure that you have good control before you conceive. Some people have difficulty in achieving this degree of control, however hard they try. It is important to understand that the risks to the baby increase as the HbA_{1c} rises and that the closer you get to 7.5% the lower the risk.

All women planning a pregnancy are advised to take supplements of folic acid (a type of vitamin) which reduces the risk of spina bifida. The dose of folic acid recommended for women with diabetes is larger than that advised for those without diabetes. You need to start taking 5 mg of folic acid daily before you try to conceive and your doctor will be able to prescribe this for you.

Good control is also needed for the rest of the pregnancy because the development and growth of the baby can be disturbed by poor

MORECAMBE BAY HOSPITALS NHS TRUST

control. In particular, the baby grows faster than normal and is large in size. If the baby has to be delivered early because it is big, it will be premature and therefore at risk of the many problems that can affect premature babies.

I have read that mothers with diabetes are more likely to have babies with congenital malformations. I am thinking of a pregnancy but am terrified of having a child with an abnormality. What can I do to prevent this?

It is true that there is an association between diabetes in the mother and congenital abnormalities in her baby. We know that the most important factor influencing this is the control of the diabetes. If the HbA_{1c} is less than 7.5% at conception, the risk of congenital abnormalities is similar to that of mothers without diabetes. The higher the HbA_{1c}, the greater the risk to the development of the baby. Therefore the best thing for you to do is to make sure that your diabetes is well controlled before you conceive.

Some women with diabetes take regular medication to protect them from kidney and heart disease. These drugs can cause damage to the baby and should be stopped before you conceive. If you are uncertain about your medication you should discuss this with your doctor.

There is good evidence that taking folic acid supplements before conception protects against abnormalities such as spina bifida, and in people with diabetes the higher dose of 5 mg is recommended. Your doctor will prescribe this for you.

All pregnant women are offered a blood test known as the triple test to screen for abnormalities such as Down's syndrome and spina bifida. This is carried out at 16 weeks and if abnormal, further tests will be offered to identify the problem. If these confirm an abnormality, your doctors will discuss the implications with you, and you may decide to have a termination.

Women with diabetes are also offered an abnormality scan at 20 weeks and this may be followed up with a detailed cardiac scan to identify any heart problems. If an abnormality is detected this will be discussed with you and a termination may be offered.

I have read that the babies of mothers with diabetes tend to be fat and have lung trouble shortly after birth and also there is a risk of hypoglycaemia. Is this true, and if so why does it happen?

We know that if the mother runs a high blood glucose during pregnancy, glucose crosses the placenta into the baby's circulation and causes the baby to become fat. This is because the baby's pancreas produces insulin even though the mother's cannot and the insulin converts the glucose into fat. As a result, the baby grows bigger during pregnancy and delivery has to be carried out early to avoid a difficult labour. If the mother is induced very early, there is a risk that she will not be ready to go into labour and the induction will fail, making a Caesarean section necessary. One of the complications of early delivery is that the baby's lungs may not be fully matured and this can lead to a condition known as respiratory distress syndrome (RDS). Babies with this condition need to be treated on a ventilator in the Special Care Baby Unit until their lungs are mature enough to cope.

If an early delivery is planned, most units give the mother a steroid injection prior to delivery. This helps to mature the baby's lungs and reduces the risk of RDS. The downside is that the steroids put up the blood glucose level and extra insulin will be needed for a couple of days until the effect of the steroids wears off.

If the mother's blood glucose levels are kept strictly within normal limits during pregnancy, babies are less likely to grow faster than normal and pregnancy can continue until the normal full term of 40 weeks. This avoids the risk of Caesarean section in the majority of women and RDS is rarely seen because the babies are fully mature.

Low blood glucose (hypoglycaemia) during the first few hours after birth occurs because the baby's pancreas has been producing excess amounts of insulin during the pregnancy to cover the high blood glucose levels which cross the placenta from the mother. If the mother's blood glucose is strictly controlled during pregnancy and delivery, hypoglycaemia in the baby is much less of a problem. It is normal practice to check the baby's blood glucose level when it is born and over the next 24 hours so that treatment can be given if the baby's glucose is low.

My baby was born with jaundice. Are babies of mothers with diabetes more likely to have this?

Yes, babies born to mothers with diabetes are more likely to be jaundiced. This is partly because they tend to be born early, but sometimes a full-term baby can become jaundiced. The reason for this is not clear but the problem is usually mild and if necessary the jaundice can be cleared with treatment.

I developed toxaemia during my last pregnancy and had to spend several weeks in hospital even though control of my diabetes was immaculate. Luckily everything turned out all right and I now have a beautiful healthy son. Was the toxaemia related to me having diabetes? Is it likely to recur in future pregnancies?

Women with diabetes are more prone to toxaemia (pre-eclampsia). You are not more likely to develop toxaemia in your future pregnancies – indeed the risk is less than in your first pregnancy.

During my last pregnancy I had 'hydramnios' and my obstetrician said that this was because I had diabetes. Is this true? And is there anything that I can do to avoid it happening in any future pregnancies?

Hydramnios is an excessive amount of fluid surrounding the baby and it is more common in mothers with diabetes. It is related to how strictly you control your diabetes throughout pregnancy. Our advice is that you can reduce the risk to an absolute minimum in future pregnancies by aiming to keep your HbA$_{1c}$ and blood glucose levels as close to normal as possible from the beginning of pregnancy (see questions on p. 194).

During the recent delivery of my fourth child (which went very smoothly) I had an insulin pump into a vein during labour. I had not had this in my previous three pregnancies, despite having diabetes. Why did I need the pump this time?

We now know that it is very important to keep your blood glucose within normal limits during labour to minimise the risk of your baby developing a low blood glucose (hypoglycaemia) in the first few hours after birth. This is most effectively and easily done using an intravenous insulin infusion combined with some glucose given as an intravenous drip. Using this method, your blood glucose can be kept strictly regulated at the normal level until your baby has been delivered. It also ensures that if any complications arise, an anaesthetic can be given without further preparation.

My first child was delivered by Caesarean section. Do I have to have a Caesarean section with my next pregnancy?

It depends why you had the Caesarean section. If it was performed for an obstetric reason that is likely to be present in the next pregnancy, the answer is yes. If it was performed because the first baby was large or just because you have diabetes, the answer could be no.

Some doctors do consider it safer to deliver a woman by Caesarean section if she has had a Caesarean section before. Others would allow you a 'trial of labour'. In other words, you would start labour and, if everything was satisfactory, you would be able to deliver your baby in the normal way.

My doctor tells me that I will have to have a Caesarean section because my baby is in a bad position and a little large. What sort of anaesthetic is best?

Nowadays approximately 50% of women who need a Caesarean section have an epidural rather than a general anaesthetic. If you have an epidural your legs and abdomen are made completely numb by injecting local anaesthetic solution through a needle into your lower back. You remain awake for the birth of your baby and therefore remember this important event. In most cases an epidural is preferred because your baby receives none of the anaesthetic and therefore is not sleepy.

If you are interested in having your baby this way, you should discuss it with your obstetrician.

My baby had difficulty with breathing in his first few days in the Special Care Baby Unit. They said this was because my control of my diabetes was poor – why was this?

It sounds as if your baby had what is called respiratory distress syndrome (RDS) which occurs most commonly in premature babies and was discussed in an earlier question. It occurs in babies of mothers with diabetes where the baby has grown too quickly because of the mother's poor blood glucose control, and requires a premature delivery. It used to be a serious threat to the babies of mothers with diabetes but now it is much less common. This is because of advances in neonatal care and better control of diabetes in pregnancy resulting in fewer premature deliveries.

If there is a possibility that your baby may be born prematurely, treatment with a steroid injection can help your baby's lungs to mature. Unfortunately the steroids can upset diabetes control for about 48 hours and you will need to be in hospital for close supervision at this time.

8 | Diabetes in the young

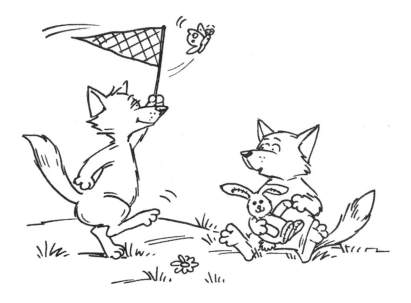

This chapter about diabetes in young people divides naturally into three main age groups: babies, children and adolescents. The sections on babies and children consist of questions asked by parents and the answers are naturally directed at them. The section on adolescents is for both young people and their parents.

Apart from the experience of Diabetes UK camps, neither of the authors has actually lived with the daily problems of bringing up a child with diabetes. However, we have listened to hundreds of parents who have felt the despair of finding that their child has diabetes and have gone on to overcome their fears and allow their child to grow up normally. Mothers and fathers usually end up being especially proud of children who have coped with the demands of diabetes.

THE BABY WITH DIABETES

My baby developed diabetes when she was four weeks old. She is now six weeks old and looks very healthy but I would like advice on how to protect her life in an emergency. What food and treatment should I give her?

Your baby probably has a very rare form of diabetes, which has only recently been identified. In 2006 research workers in Exeter and Oxford discovered that babies diagnosed under the age of six months usually have a form of diabetes which does not need treatment with insulin. Like your little girl, most of these children are diagnosed at the age of 4 to 6 weeks and they have a condition called neonatal diabetes, which can be confirmed by genetic testing. If these tests are positive, her diabetes should be controlled by a drug called glibenclamide, which is available in liquid form and can be added to her feeds. Many cases of neonatal diabetes clear up on their own within the first year, while others can be treated with glibenclamide in the long term.

My little boy is nearly 12 months old and has been ill for a month, losing weight and always crying. Diabetes has just been diagnosed. Does this mean injections for life?

Yes. Unfortunately it does literally mean injections for life as there is no other form of treatment at present. However, alternative methods of giving insulin are being explored and other areas of research, including islet cell transplants, look promising, so it is possible that there will be an alternative to insulin injections in your child's lifetime. For more information about current research see Chapter 10.

The thought of having to stick needles repeatedly into a young child can be horrifying to parents. There are ways of making injections less threatening, such as playing games in which you inject a teddy bear (using a different needle) or yourself (without insulin).

You should be able to devise some rewards which will help your son accept injections as part of his normal day. Parents of young children may find the treatment more upsetting than the child does himself, as he has grown up knowing no other way of life. Encourage your child to help at injection time by getting the equipment ready or perhaps by pushing in the button on the pen and pulling out the needle.

How can I collect urine for testing from my 18-month-old son? I have been given lots of different suggestions but none of them seem to work.

In the past, urine tests were the only way to see if diabetes was under control, and as you point out, it could be difficult to obtain a sample of urine. Fortunately, we now have meters which operate with very small samples of blood, so it is much easier to check the blood glucose. The only time you need to test urine is when your child is ill and you need to check for ketones. Many infants will produce a specimen by reflex into a small potty when undressed. You can also squeeze a wet nappy directly onto a urine testing stick.

Ketostix® or Ketur Test® are used to test for ketones. Infants are much more likely than older people to have ketones in the urine because when fasting, they rapidly switch their source of energy from carbohydrate to fat, resulting in ketone production. You should not worry if ketones are present in small amounts on one occasion; if they persist and your son is unwell, you should contact the hospital team.

I have been told by the hospital nurse that I must prick my little girl's finger to check her blood glucose. She is four years old and has just been found to have diabetes. I can see the importance of insulin injections, but do I really need to keep pricking her finger?

Unfortunately, at the present time, blood testing is the only method we have to help decide how much insulin is required. Parents naturally dislike causing their children pain but with the minute amounts of blood needed for modern meters, blood tests are surprisingly well accepted by young children. These tests are particularly important if your daughter looks or feels unwell, as they are the only reliable way of deciding whether she is hypo or just tired and hungry. Your hospital team will be able to recommend a finger pricker suitable for your child. Details of finger prickers and small volume blood glucose meters are given in Table 4.2. It may help to speak to other parents of children with diabetes.

> *My 2-year-old daughter has diabetes and makes an awful fuss about food. Meals are turning into a regular struggle. Have you any suggestions?*

Food is of great emotional significance to all children. If meals are eaten without complaint, then everyone will be happy. However, all children go through phases of food refusal because of a need to assert their independence, manipulate a situation or just wind up their parents. In most families, mealtimes can become a battleground at some stage and the only way for you to win is to remain in control of the weapon. Usually when young children begin this phase (at 10–18 months), they dislike being told to leave the table and go away. They often return and eat rather than remain alone and hungry.

The battle is even more difficult for parents of a child with diabetes – your daughter also has some explosive weapons! However, you must stay in control: try to maintain a relaxed approach to eating and distract her attention away from food with toys, music or stories. If the relaxed approach fails and she refuses to eat properly, you may have to resort to sending her away from the table until she is hungry enough to give in. If you feel anxious about her becoming hypo, wait until you see what she has eaten before you decide how much insulin to give. Be prepared to modify the type of carbohydrate within reason if she consistently refuses the sort of food recommended by the specialist team. Bread, potatoes, biscuits, fruit juices and even ice-cream can be offered as alternative choices.

Susie Orbach has recently written an excellent book called *On eating.* Figure 8.1 reprints advice given in the *Guardian* (reproduced with permission from AP Watt Ltd on behalf of Susie Orbach).

THE CHILD WITH DIABETES

Since my 6-year-old daughter was found to have diabetes, I have felt very isolated and although the hospital diabetes team has been very supportive, I would love to be able to talk to somebody who has been through the same experience. How can I make contact with other parents?

Many voluntary groups of Diabetes UK have a Parents' section which organises activities for children with diabetes and their families. They also allow parents to support each other. Alternatively you could ask your hospital diabetes team to help you make contact with other parents.

My 5-year-old son has had diabetes since he was 18 months and he is only 96 cm (3 ft 2 in) tall. I have been told that he is very short for his age. The doctor says that poorly controlled diabetes could be slowing his growth. Is this true?

The average height for a 5-year-old boy is 108 cm (3 ft 6 in), so your son is certainly short for his age. If he has had high glucose levels over a period of months, this could slow his growth. If you can manage to keep his diabetes under control and make sure that he has plenty to eat, he should grow rapidly and may even catch up with his normal height. However, his short stature may be due to a growth disorder and may need further investigation. Speak to your specialist team about this.

Figure 8.1

FOOD AND YOUR CHILDREN

Dos and don'ts for babies and toddlers

- Do introduce your baby and toddler to the mashed-up version of the foods and tastes you relish, including the herbs and spices.

- Do clip a baby seat on to the table if possible so that the baby can be part of family eating and have her interest in what you are eating stimulated.

- Do respect your baby or toddler when they say 'no'. When they turn away from eating, offer them some other food and if it doesn't hit the spot, allow them to stop eating. They will soon let you know if they are hungry again.

- Do let your baby and toddler muck about with food and make a mess. Food is a source of creativity as well as fuel.

- Don't encourage them to eat five more spoonfuls for Grandma, or the starving children elsewhere, or play games that trick them into eating. Show them your relish in food.

Dos and don'ts for primary-age children

- Do put lots of different kinds of food out and let the children choose what they fancy.

- Don't differentiate between kids' and adult food. Children's tastes will be as complex and sophisticated as the foods they are exposed to.

- Do value foods equally so that broccoli becomes no less of a special food than ice-cream.

- Do let children see you stopping when you are full and leaving food on your plate.

- Do let children leave food when they've had enough or when they are compelled to rush off to do something more interesting than eat. If you are worried they have not had enough to eat, make sure there is food around for them to come back and refuel on.

- Don't ever reward them for eating their greens by offering them sweets or ice-cream or cake. Do let them eat in whatever order they like including having dessert first if they are desperate for the carbohydrates.

- Don't cheer them up or jolly them out of a sad or angry mood with food unless you know they are hungry. Do let them tell you how they feel without shushing them or humouring them out of their upset. If they tell you and get their feelings out in the open, the pain will dissipate faster.

Dos and don'ts for adolescents

- Do expect them to eat fast food. It's a sign of independence, of showing how different they are from you, of making it with their peers. If you've fed them interesting food all along, don't despair, they won't be able to eat junk every day.

- Do sit together around the table several nights a week. If they've stocked up on food after school and aren't hungry, let them sit with you while you eat so that they get accustomed to being around food and only eating it when they are hungry.

- Don't have fights while eating together. It fuses food and conflict together.

- Do have tons of food in the house and expect erratic eating. Teenagers have fast metabolisms and many need to eat lots more than adults.

- Do tolerate their cooking even if their experiments violate your basic principles in the kitchen.

- Do discourage them from dieting. Set the example by never doing it yourself.

- Don't have a corner for 'junk' food. Disperse it among the foods you consider good.

I have been told not to expect my daughter to be as tall as she would have been had she not had diabetes. Is this true? If so, what can I do to help her reach her maximum height?

Unless your daughter's diabetes control has been very poor, there is no reason why she should not reach her proper height without any special encouragement. Diabetes will not necessarily stunt her growth but it could if her blood glucose control is not good.

My 6-year-old daughter has had diabetes for four years. She is on 12 units of Novomix 30 insulin twice a day. Her morning blood glucose is always 4–8 mmol/L but her tests are more than 15 mmol/L at bedtime. We are getting different advice from different people. What do you advise?

This problem is often seen in people having premixed insulin. The mixture contains enough long-acting insulin to provide overnight background insulin but not enough short-acting insulin for her evening meal. The usual solution to this common problem requires an extra injection of insulin and you may feel that your little girl is not ready for this. If she were to 'split the evening dose' by having short-acting insulin analogue before her meal and some long-acting insulin when she goes to bed, the doses of each of these can be adjusted independently so her blood glucose is normal both at bedtime and on waking.

My son, aged 10, started insulin last year and his dose has gradually dropped. Now he has come off insulin completely and is on diet alone. Will he now be off insulin permanently?

No. There is a 99.9% chance that he will have to go back on insulin eventually. This so-called 'honeymoon period' (see the section *Dosage* in Chapter 3) can be very unsettling as it raises hopes that the diabetes has cleared up. Unfortunately, this never happens in young people and he is likely to need insulin again within 12 months.

Are there any special schools for children with diabetes?

There are no special schools for children with diabetes and we do not think they would be a good idea. It is important that young people with diabetes grow up in normal surroundings and are not encouraged to regard themselves as 'different'. Children with diabetes should go to normal schools and grow up in a normal family atmosphere.

I think my newly-diagnosed son is using his insulin injections as a way of avoiding school. I can't send him to school unless he has his insulin but it sometimes takes ages before I can get him to have his injection. I have two younger children and a husband whom I also have to help to get to school and work. How should I cope with my temperamental son?

You raise several related points. You assume that he is using his insulin injections to avoid school, and you may be right, especially if he resisted going to school before developing diabetes. In this case you should try the same tactics that you used before. Alternatively, his dislike of school could be related to the diabetes, for example an overprotective attitude by sports instructors, frequent hypos or embarrassment about eating snacks between meals. If you suspect such difficulties, a talk to your son and his teacher might clear the air.

Another possibility is that rather than trying to avoid school, he is actually frightened of his insulin injections so that things get off to a slow start in the morning. A clue to this might be his willingness to take his evening insulin injection. If this is also a drawn out process, the problem probably lies with his dislike of injections, rather than school. For some children, injections become the focus of their rejection of the burden of diabetes: by delaying their injection, they fight their diabetes. The specialist paediatric team will be keen to help with this problem and they may also put you in touch with other parents who have experience of similar situations.

Diabetes UK has produced a pack called Information for Schools and Youth Organizations to help parents communicate with the school. It contains information to be given to teachers and those responsible for children with diabetes. You can contact Diabetes UK (the address is in Appendix 2) for a copy of this publication.

When my son starts school, would it be better for him to return home for lunch or should we let him eat school dinners?

It depends largely on your son's temperament and attitude to school. Some 4-year-olds take to school very well and are happy to stay there all day, while others take time to settle in the new environment. They may be happier to go home for lunch, particularly if they dislike the food served up at school. It is important that your son eats a proper lunch and whether or not he likes the school meals may be the deciding factor. It would be best to ask the advice of his teachers and make sure that someone will take the responsibility of choosing suitable food for your son – you can't leave that to a child of four or five. The diabetes specialist nurse will be happy to liaise with the school.

My 10-year-old son has recently been diagnosed with diabetes. What is the best age for him to start doing his own injections?

The fear of injections may loom large in a child's view of his own diabetes, but in fact many children make less fuss if they do their own injections and most diabetes specialist nurses would encourage a 10-year-old to do his own injections from day one. However, all children are different and there is no correct age for children to take responsibility for their own injections. Some children need a break from injecting themselves from time to time and might ask a parent to do it for them. If there is an injection problem, you should discuss this with the diabetes specialist team who will be experienced in dealing with this difficulty.

Some children may benefit from going on a Diabetes UK holiday, where they will see other children taking insulin with confidence. You will find details in *Balance* or on the Diabetes UK website.

I am a junior school teacher and have a child with diabetes in my class. I have read up all I can about diabetes. Most of my questions have been answered but I cannot discover what to do if the child eats too much sugar. Will he go into a coma? If so, what do I do then?

Eating sugar or sweets may make his blood glucose rise, in which case he may feel thirsty and generally off-colour. Coma from a high blood glucose takes hours or even days to develop and there is only cause for concern if he becomes very drowsy or starts vomiting. If this does happen, you should contact his parents. A child who is vomiting with poor diabetes control probably needs to go to hospital.

The most common sort of coma, which may occur over a matter of ten minutes, is due to a hypo. This often shows itself as irritable behaviour and mental confusion. In this case the blood glucose level is too low and he needs to be given sugar *at once*. He should return to normal within about ten minutes. The causes of hypo are delayed meals, missed snacks or extra exercise. If there is any doubt about whether his condition is caused by a high or a low blood glucose, it is always safer to give some sugar as this will correct a hypo but will not make a high blood glocose significantly worse. Refer to the list of symptoms in Chapter 12. If you need to send him elsewhere for treatment of low blood glucose (such as to the school nurse) make sure he is accompanied.

The diabetes paediatric nurse will know your pupil and would be in a position to help with advice.

Can I apply for an allowance to look after my son who has frequent hypos and needs a lot of extra care?

Yes, as the parent of a child with unstable diabetes you can apply for a Disability Living Allowance, which is a non-means tested benefit. Many people in your position have successfully applied and feel that it provides some recognition of the burden of being responsible for a child with diabetes, especially if hypos are a major problem. There is more information about Social Security benefits in Chapter 5.

There is an opposing view that diabetes should not be regarded as a disability and that applying for an allowance fosters a feeling that the child is an invalid. This is an individual decision.

My little boy has diabetes and is always having coughs and colds. These make him very ill and he always becomes very sugary during each illness despite antibiotics from the doctor. Could you please give me some guidelines for coping with his diabetes during these infections?

Minor illnesses can certainly upset diabetes control and if your son's blood glucose is high, this will make him feel even more unwell. You should follow the guidelines in Figure 8.2.

I am head teacher of a school for deaf children and one of my pupils developed diabetes two years ago. Since then his learning ability has deteriorated. Can this have any connection with his diabetes?

No. Diabetes in itself has no effect on learning ability and there are plenty of children with diabetes who excel academically. Poorly controlled diabetes with a very high blood glucose could reduce his powers of concentration, however. Hypoglycaemic attacks are usually short lasting but he could be missing a few key items while his blood glucose is low and be unable to catch up.

At a psychological level, the double handicap of deafness and diabetes could be affecting his morale and self-confidence. Perhaps he would be helped by meeting other boys of his age who also have diabetes. This often helps children to realise that diabetes is compatible with normal life and activities. Contact the paediatric diabetes team responsible for your pupil or failing that approach Diabetes UK.

My son was recently awarded a scholarship to a well-known public school but when they found he had diabetes, he was refused admission on medical grounds. They can give no positive reason for this and our consultant has tried very hard to make them change their minds. Why should he be so penalised?

This was a disgraceful decision based on prejudice. It would be worth discussing this with Diabetes UK who are looking for examples of discrimination against people with diabetes. The Disability Discrimination Act applies to education and you could consider seeking legal advice. However, you may question whether you would want your son to go to a school which takes this attitude to diabetes.

Should my son tell his school friends about his diabetes?

It is very important that your son tells his close friends that he has diabetes. He should explain about hypos and tell them that, if he does behave in an odd way, they should make him take sugar. He will need to show them where he keeps his supplies of glucose. If your son shows his friends how he measures his blood glucose, they will probably be interested in diabetes and be keen to help him with it. Some young people like to bring a friend to their clinic appointments. As he becomes older and spends more time out and about with his friends, he will naturally involve them more in his diabetes.

Figure 8.2 When your child is unwell

Extra units of insulin required depending on blood glucose level					
Total daily units of insulin	BG less than 13 mmol/L with or without ketones	BG 13–22 mmol/L without ketones	BG 13–22 mmol/L with ketones	BG over 23 mmol/L without ketones	BG over 23 mmol/L with ketones
1–10 per day	Normal dose	1u before each meal and before bed	2u before each meal and before bed	2u before each meal and before bed	6u before each meal and before bed
11–20 per day	Normal dose	2u before each meal and before bed	4u before each meal and before bed	4u before each meal and before bed	2u before each meal and before bed
21–49 per day	Normal dose	4u before each meal and before bed	6u before each meal and before bed	6u before each meal and before bed	8u before each meal and before bed
50 plus per day	Normal dose	8u before each meal and before bed	10u before each meal and before bed	10u before each meal and before bed	12u before each meal and before bed

• Insulin should always be given. If your child is vomiting, and has low blood glucose, the dose of insulin may need to be reduced (see **Hypos** below). Be sure to check four hours later and give extra insulin if it is high. If in doubt, contact your hospital diabetes team for advice.

• If your child uses Humalog, NovoRapid or Humulin S insulin separately from long-acting insulin, the extra units should be given in this form. Otherwise, you should give the extra units from your usual mix of insulin.

- **Vomiting**

  Replace carbohydrate foods with sugary drinks, such as iced lemon barley water (1 glass taken over one hour).

  If fluids are not tolerated over the course of one hour or if your child is persistently vomiting for half an hour, you should seek medical help. Make direct contact with the hospital specialist team or your GP.

- **High blood glucose**

  If your child has blood glucose over 13 mmol/L for two consecutive readings and feels unwell, the blood glucose should be monitored at least four times per day and the guidelines for extra units of insulin should be followed.

  If your child has high blood glucose, but has no appetite, you should replace the carbohydrate foods with sugary drinks to avoid hypos.

  If you have urine testing strips for ketones, the urine should be tested at least four times per day, noting the time of testing. If ketones are present in the urine, follow the guidelines for extra units of insulin and contact your hospital specialist team or GP for advice. Ketones suggest that the body is short of insulin.

  Extra units of insulin should be given until the blood glucose is below 13 mmol/L.

- **Hypos**

  If your child does not want to eat and the blood glucose is less than 7, you may need to reduce the dose of insulin to avoid hypos. During the illness, you should check the blood glucose at least four times a day.

  Adapted from the Northampton General Hospital guidelines and Diabetes UK 'Coping with illness'.

My 10-year-old son moves on to a large comprehensive school in a few months' time. Up until now he has been in a small junior school where all the staff know about his diabetes. I worry that he will be swamped in the 'big' school where he will come across lots of different teachers who know nothing about his condition. Have you any advice on this problem?

Moving up to a big comprehensive school is always a daunting experience and is bound to cause the parents of a child with diabetes extra worry. It is important to talk to your son's form teacher, preferably before the first day of term when he or she will have hundreds of new problems to cope with. Assume that the teacher knows nothing about diabetes.

- Make sure that they know your child needs daily insulin injections.

- Warn them he may need to eat a snack during a lesson to ward off a hypo.

- Describe how your son behaves when hypo and emphasise the importance of giving him sugar. If he needs to go somewhere else for treatment of the hypo, he must be accompanied.

- Staggered lunchtimes may be a problem as he may need to eat at a fixed time each day.

- If he needs a lunchtime injection, you should make his teachers aware of this and agree how he should store and access his insulin, pen device and blood testing equipment.

- You will need to be told if he is going to be kept in late (e.g. for detention) as he may need to eat at the end of the school day.

- Ask his class teacher to make sure all your son's other teachers know these facts.

The hospital diabetes nurse will be pleased to visit the school to reinforce these points. Diabetes UK supplies a School Pack, which provides written information for teachers. It is especially important to speak personally to his sports and swimming instructors so they are aware of the possibility of a hypo. You will probably have to repeat this exercise at the beginning of every school year.

What arrangements can I make with school about my 9-year-old daughter's special requirements for school dinners?

It is important to go and see the head teacher and preferably the caterer to explain that your daughter must have her dinner on time. Explain that she needs a certain amount of carbohydrate in a form that she will eat and that she should avoid puddings containing sugar. Most clinics have a diabetes specialist nurse or health visitor, who could go to the school and give advice.

Most parents of children with diabetes get round the whole problem by providing a packed lunch. This gives you more control over what your daughter eats and you can supply the sort of food she likes.

When she goes on to secondary school she may be faced with a cafeteria system. This should allow her to choose suitable food, but of course there is a risk that she will choose unsuitable items. Recently there has been pressure on schools to provide healthy food, which should be a help for your daughter.

My son has diabetes. Can I allow him to go on school trips?

In general the answer is yes, but for your own peace of mind you need to be satisfied that one of the staff on the trip will take responsibility for your son. Day trips should be no problem as long as someone can be sure that he eats on time and has his insulin injections if necessary. At junior school level, long trips away from home, especially on the continent, could be more difficult and it really depends whether you can find a member of staff whom you trust. They will need to keep an eye on your son and to know how to cope with problems like a bad hypo. Once in secondary school most children manage to go away on trips with the school, scouts or a youth group. Of course one of the adults in the party should be responsible, but as your son gets older he will be better able to look after himself. Diabetes UK has the following checklist for things to take on school trips and holidays:

- identification necklace or bracelet;
- glucose;
- insulin, insulin pen, needles;
- equipment for testing blood glucose;
- food to cover journeys with extra for unexpected delays;
- Glucogel®.

This is part of the Information for Schools and Youth Organizations Pack, which is available from Diabetes UK.

My 12-year-old son has diabetes with rather erratic control. We have heard about DAFNE, an education programme which is said to be wonderful. Is there a DAFNE for children?

The DAFNE programme (see p. 91) is an effective form of education for adults with Type 1 diabetes. It depends on people working in a group with skilled educators. With financial backing from Diabetes UK, a new DAFNE course is being designed for children aged 11–16. Children, parents and teachers have been involved in planning this programme and it is now being tried out in six centres in the UK.

My 10-year-old child has heard about Diabetes UK camps from the clinic. I am a bit worried about letting him go off on his own for two weeks. Do you not think that I should wait a few years before sending him to a camp?

No, he's not too young to go. Diabetes UK has been running holidays for children since the 1930s and this remains a core activity of the organisation. Young children enjoy group holidays, and gain a sense of confidence from being with other children with diabetes – for once they are not the odd ones out. The children learn from each other and from the staff. Your son will have an exciting holiday and you will have a few weeks off from the responsibility of looking after his diabetes.

My daughter would like to go on a Diabetes UK camp. Could you tell me something about the arrangements?

The Care team of Diabetes UK has many years experience in running holidays for children. The average camp consists of 30–35 children who are supervised by the following staff:

- warden, responsible for planning;
- 1–2 deputy wardens;
- senior medical officer, who is experienced in diabetes;
- junior medical officer;
- 2–4 nurses, usually with a special interest in diabetes;
- 3 dictitians;
- 8 junior leaders, young adults with diabetes themselves, who give up their time to help.

The staff-to-child ratio is about 1:2 and there is always close supervision on outings and all sports, especially swimming.

These educational holidays provide valuable experience and require a large number of helpers. Although Diabetes UK tries to keep down the costs, some people may be put off by the price. If you are worried about meeting the cost of the holiday, your local voluntary group of Diabetes UK may be able to help.

DIABETES AND THE ADOLESCENT

My 16-year-old son is only 157 cm tall (5 ft 2 in) and very immature. I have heard that children with diabetes reach puberty a year or two later than anyone else. Will he grow later?

If your son is sexually underdeveloped, he will certainly have a growth spurt when he goes into puberty. However, his height is under average for a boy of 16. His growth could have been affected by poor diabetes control but there are other possible factors, including the height of his father and yourself. If you are both a normal height, you should consult your clinic doctor rather than assuming it is due to his diabetes.

My daughter and I are getting extremely anxious although our GP tells us there is nothing to worry about. She developed diabetes when she was 14 years old, one year after her periods had started. They stopped completely with the diabetes and have never started again, although we have now waited for two years. Is our GP right to be calm and patient, or are we right to be worried?

A major upset to the system such as diabetes may cause periods to stop for a while but it is unusual for this to last as long as two years unless her control is poor or she is very thin. After this length of time your daughter should probably be seen by an endocrinologist and you should speak to your GP about this.

I am nearly 15 and have not started my periods. Is this because I have diabetes? Since I was diagnosed, I have put on a lot of weight.

On average, girls with diabetes tend to start their periods at an older age. We assume from your question that you are now overweight and this may be another cause for delay in menstruation.

Provided there are other signs of puberty such as breast development and growth of pubic hair, you should try to lose weight and control your diabetes carefully. If you have still not seen a period by the time you are 16, you should discuss the matter with your specialist team.

My son will be going to university next year. While we are all delighted and proud of him, I worry because he will be living away from home for the first time. Since he was diagnosed seven years ago, I have taken most of the responsibility, including the practical arrangements of his meals. My son has done his best to ignore his diabetes and I wonder how he will cope with this on his own.

If your son has got into university, he should be able to look after his diabetes. However, you are right to point out that his attitude to diabetes is also important. All mothers worry when their children leave home for the first time and it is natural for a child with diabetes to cause extra worry. Most children like to spread their wings when first leaving home and you can expect a period of adjustment to his new responsibilities. Provided that he realises why good control of his diabetes is important, he should become more responsible in time. It would be a good idea for your son to contact the diabetes clinic in his university town, so they can give any support he might need. Your own paediatric team would be able to make this introduction.

How does diabetes affect my chances of finding a partner?

The short answer is that diabetes should not affect your chances of finding a partner in any way. However, if you have had the experience of being rejected because of diabetes, this is likely to have a bad effect on your self-confidence. This in turn may make it more difficult for you to approach a potential partner in a positive way. You must remember that diabetes is nothing to be ashamed of. Most partners are very supportive and will want to know how they can help you to look after your diabetes.

I have recently met a boy who I'm really keen on, but am frightened that he will be put off if I tell him I have diabetes. What should I do?

The standard answer is that you must tell your new boyfriend at the beginning. However, you must be reluctant to do this or you would not be asking the question. There is no need to broadcast the fact that you have diabetes but if you get to know each other well, there will come a time when it will feel natural to tell him. If he is close to you, he will want to know everything about you and will probably wish to be involved in your diabetes.

My 15-year-old son developed diabetes at the age of 12. Initially he was very sensible about his diabetes but recently he has become resentful, saying that he is different from everyone else and blaming us for his disease. What do you suggest?

People of all ages feel resentful at some stage about the major impact that diabetes has on their life. Many 12-year-old children conform with their parents' wishes and generally do as they are told. However, by the age of 15 other important pressures are beginning to influence a young person. Teenagers usually have a tumult of emotions and hormonal changes, which mean that diabetes is unlikely to be at the top of their priority list. While as parents you will be happy to make allowances for diabetes, for example by providing special meals, most young lads want to be part of the gang and hate to appear 'different'.

At a diabetes camp for young leaders, which was restricted to hand-picked, well adjusted young adults with diabetes, the organisers were surprised to discover how angry the young people felt about their condition. Of course this anger will often be directed at the parents. We will try to give some general advice which should apply to most adolescent problems:

- Keep lines of communication open;

- Boost his self-esteem by giving praise where praise is due even if your own self-esteem is taking a hammering;

- Allow your son to make his own decisions about diabetes; if you force him to comply, he may simply avoid confrontation by deceiving you;

- Remind yourself that adolescence does not last for ever and is an important part of growing up;

- Try to make contact with other parents of teenagers with diabetes. They may have some useful insights and come up with a new approach. The local voluntary group of Diabetes UK should be able to put you in touch with other people in the same situation.

The paediatric specialist team will have experience in these issues and may be able to give advice.

Our 15-year-old daughter has had diabetes for four years and until recently has always been well controlled. Now it is very difficult to get her to take an interest in her diabetes and she has stopped doing blood tests. At the last clinic visit, the doctor said that her HbA$_{1c}$ was very high and he thought she was probably missing some of her injections. I really do not know what to do.

This is a very upsetting situation for all concerned and unfortunately it is a common scenario. Diabetes is hard because it places great demands and restrictions on people but in the short term they have nothing to show for their efforts. It is very common for people to avoid the prescribed treatment and the reasons for this are very complex. Like most girls of her age, your daughter probably wants to lose weight and she may have discovered that allowing her glucose levels to run high by missing some insulin injections is an effective way of getting her weight down quickly.

There is no easy solution to this problem especially as many girls in this situation turn up at the clinic and announce brightly that every-

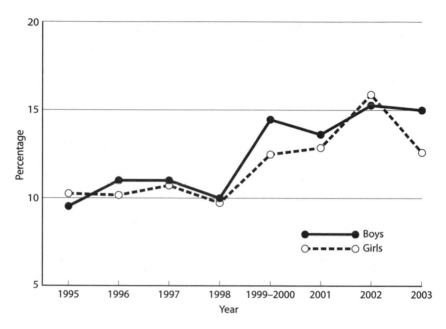

Figure 8.3 Obesity trends among children aged 2–15,
England, by sex 1995–2003

Jotangia D, Moody A, Stamatakis E, Wardle H (2005) *Obesity among children under 11,*
London: National Centre for Social Research, Department of Epidemiology and Public Health
at the Royal Free and University College Medical School

thing is fine. Simply challenging your daughter and threatening her with the long-term complications of diabetes is unlikely to help and will probably create a barrier between you. It is better to try and get her to realise that you understand that living with diabetes is not easy, and allow her to express her own feelings about it. Of course she may be at a stage of feeling that parents are light-years away from her own experience, in which case she is more likely to unburden herself to a close friend, especially someone else with diabetes.

If you are feeling upset by the doctor's suggestion, you should probably talk to one of the specialist nurses in the paediatric team.

My nephew, who is 11 years old, has just been found to have diabetes but has been started on tablets. I thought that all young people with diabetes had to take insulin injections.

Until recently, nearly all children with diabetes fell into the Type 1 group and therefore needed insulin treatment from the time of diagnosis. In the last few years, however, Type 2 diabetes has become increasingly common in children. This increase in Type 2 diabetes in the young is more advanced in the USA, where in some children's clinics more than half the children have Type 2 diabetes. This increase is related to changes in lifestyle of the population in general and young people in particular. To put it bluntly, the epidemic of obesity is the result of eating too much and taking very little exercise. Most experts feel that Europe is five to ten years behind America in the obesity epidemic (see Figures 8.3 and 8.4).

Type 2 diabetes in children should be treated in the same way as in adults. First line treatment consists of an education package, which allows the child and parents to express their fears and helps them understand what this diagnosis means and what they can do about it. At some stages of the process, siblings should be involved as they will be affected by the diagnosis and may become useful partners in support of their brother or sister. The family should be encouraged to make changes in lifestyle and, in particular, decide how they can improve their patterns of eating. It is important to be shown how to monitor blood glucose in order to assess the response to any changes they make and to discover the effect of different foodstuffs and of exercise. Like most people with Type 2 diabetes, your nephew is faced with the prospect of taking increasing numbers of tablets to control his blood glucose and at some stage he will need insulin treatment.

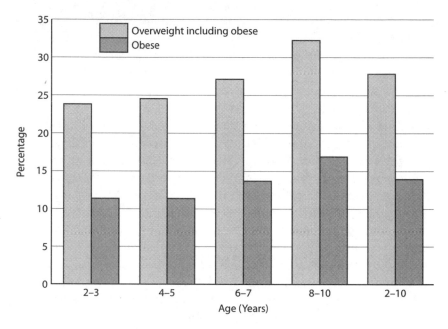

Figure 8.4 Prevalence of overweight and obesity among children, by age, England, 2003

Our 16-year-old daughter has just been found to have Type 2 diabetes. Apart from not needing insulin, are there any other differences between Type 1 and Type 2 diabetes?

It may come as a relief to be told that although your daughter has diabetes, she will not need insulin injections – at least for the time being. However, Type 2 diabetes is at least as serious a condition as Type 1. This is because young people with Type 2 diabetes, like adults with this condition, carry an extra threat of heart disease, though this will not apply to your daughter until she is much older. The risk factors include high cholesterol, triglycerides and blood pressure, and increased waist circumference.

A study in America has looked at the frequency with which these risk factors appeared in different groups of young people aged 12–19 years. In the general population of American children, 6.4% in this age range had two or more of these risk factors. In young people with Type 1 diabetes, the frequency was 14%, while in those with Type 2 diabetes it was greater than 90%.

Although this information is bound to worry you, all these risk factors can be identified and corrected. It is important that your daughter has regular checks for body weight, cholesterol and blood pressure and if these are above the normal for her age, she should receive treatment to prevent or delay the risk of heart disease as she grows older. Some drugs used for treatment of cholesterol and blood pressure should not be used in pregnancy and your daughter needs to be aware of this.

Most children with Type 2 diabetes are overweight, and if this applies to your daughter, it is essential that she cut down her calorie intake. It would be helpful for her to see a specialist dietitian.

9 | Long-term complications

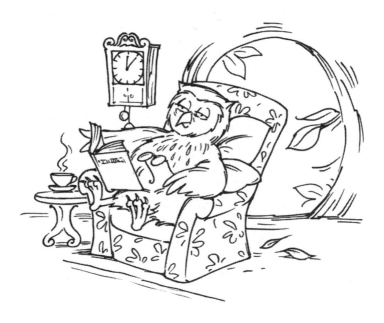

Before insulin was discovered, people with diabetes did not survive long enough to develop diabetic complications as we know them today. In the early days after the great discovery in 1922, it was widely believed that insulin cured diabetes. We are now in a better position to realise that, although insulin produced nothing short of miraculous recovery for those on the verge of death, returning them to a full and active life, it does not cure the condition. Nevertheless, if insulin is used properly to achieve good diabetes control, it is possible to have a long and healthy life.

Life expectancy has increased progressively since insulin was first introduced and there are now many thousands of people who have successfully completed more than 50 years of insulin treatment. Increased longevity has brought with it a number of the so-called 'long-term complications'. Some of these complications also occur in older people who do not have diabetes. For example heart disease, stroke and poor circulation in the legs are complications which can occur as part of the ageing process. Others are not seen in people without diabetes and these are therefore the complications specific to diabetes. The three most important are eye damage (retinopathy), nerve damage (neuropathy) and kidney damage (nephropathy).

Diabetic retinopathy can lead to loss of vision and is the most common cause of blindness registration in people under 65 in the UK. Fortunately only a small proportion of people suffer complete visual loss. Diabetic neuropathy, by leading to loss of feeling, particularly in the feet, makes people susceptible to infections and occasionally gangrene, leading to the risk of amputation. It can also cause impotence. Diabetic nephropathy can cause kidney failure and is now the most common reason for referral for renal dialysis and transplantation in young people, although the numbers are very small.

It is not surprising that people dread the thought of diabetic complications. In the past they worried but did not ask about them as they were a taboo subject. Nowadays most people expect to be fully informed about the possible risk that they face and what they can do to reduce it.

There is a great deal of misinformation circulating about diabetic complications and it is important that people receive a balanced and accurate picture.

Although medical science has made impressive progress since the discovery of insulin, there is still a long way to go. There is overwhelming scientific evidence to show that the risk of complications is directly related to blood glucose control. Thus, prevention of complications is possible by tight control of the blood glucose concentration. The evidence comes from a very large clinical trial carried out in the USA: the Diabetes Control and Complications Trial (DCCT), which provided indisputable evidence that complications can be avoided by strict blood glucose control, aiming for an HbA_{1c} of 7%. There is more information about the trials in the the introduction to Chapter 4: **Monitoring and control**.

Some of the questions in this chapter relating to eyes and feet are not strictly questions about complications, but as they do not easily fit in anywhere else in the book they have been included in this chapter under their specific headings.

GENERAL QUESTIONS

My child has had diabetes for three years and I am trying to find out more about the disease. I recently read a book which said that some people with diabetes may go blind. I don't know if this is true and find it very upsetting. Surely they shouldn't be allowed to write such things in books that young people might read?

You raise a very important matter. Diabetes was almost always fatal within one or two years of diagnosis until the outlook was revolutionised by the discovery of insulin. Nonetheless, it still required a lot of work and development of modern insulins before someone with diabetes was able to lead a relatively normal life.

After several years it became obvious that some people were developing long-term complications which took many years to develop. This became the focus of a massive research project, requiring the investment of much effort and many years of work by doctors, scientists and the 1441 people with diabetes who took part in the study, the Diabetes Control and Complications Trial (DCCT). We now understand how some of these complications occur, and we know how to treat them if they do. We realise that strict control of diabetes is important in their prevention. For this reason, all doctors and other medical personnel treating people with diabetes spend much of their time and effort trying to help them improve their control and keep their blood glucose as near normal as possible. These complications do not occur in all people by any means, although nowadays, with people living longer than ever before, the complications are becoming more important.

You ask whether facts like these should be made available to people with diabetes. The majority of people like to be correctly informed about their condition, its management and its complications. Doctors and nurses have responded to this by being much more frank in discussing all aspects of the condition. However, we agree that there is no point in frightening a young child before he is able to understand the risks and implications of diabetes.

What are the complications and what should I keep a lookout for to ensure that they are picked up as soon as possible?

The complications specific to diabetes are known as diabetic retinopathy, neuropathy and nephropathy.

- Retinopathy means damage to the retina at the back of the eye.

- Neuropathy means damage to the nerves. This can affect nerves supplying any part of the body but is generally referred to as either 'peripheral' when affecting nerves supplying muscles and skin, or as 'autonomic' when affecting nerves supplying organs such as the bladder, the bowel and the heart.

- Nephropathy is damage affecting the kidneys, which in the first instance makes them more leaky, so that albumin (protein) appears in the urine. At a later stage it may affect the function of the kidneys and in severe cases lead to kidney failure.

The best way of detecting complications early is to visit your doctor or clinic for regular review. You should have a check once a year, either at your doctor's surgery or at the hospital clinic, so any complications can be detected at a stage when they can be treated. Most areas now offer annual retinal photography to screen for diabetic eye changes. It is important to make use of this service.

Prevention is, however, clearly better than treatment and, if you can control your diabetes well, you will be less likely to suffer these complications.

I am very worried that I might develop complications after some years of having diabetes. Is it possible to avoid complications in later life? If so, how?

We believe that all people could avoid complications if they were able to control their diabetes from the day that they were diagnosed. There are now many cases on record of people who have had Type 1 diabetes for 50 years or more and are completely free from any signs of complications. Things are a bit different for Type 2 diabetes, which may be present for many years without causing any symptoms. Some people may be unfortunate enough to develop a complication, such as a foot ulcer, before diabetes itself is diagnosed.

The best advice we can give you on how to avoid complications is to take the control of your blood glucose and diabetes seriously from the outset and to attend regularly for review and supervision by somebody experienced in the management of people with diabetes. Focus on how to look after yourself in such a way that you can achieve and maintain an HbA_{1c} in the target range (6.5–7.5%) (see the section *Haemoglobin A_{1c}* in Chapter 4). If you can do that and keep your HbA_{1c} normal, you can look forward to a life free from the risk of diabetic complications.

To what extent are the complications of diabetes genetically determined?

This is a very difficult question to answer. Most specialists believe that there is a hereditary factor which predisposes some people to develop certain complications and makes others relatively immune from them. So far, scientific evidence for this is not very strong but there is a lot of work in progress in this field at the moment.

What is the life expectancy of someone with Type 1 diabetes and why?

Life expectancy in people with diabetes depends greatly on their age when the diagnosis is made. The older the person at the time of diagnosis the closer their expected life span is to that of someone who does not have diabetes.

In the past, when diabetes was diagnosed in early childhood, the life span of people with Type 1 diabetes was generally reduced, mainly because of premature deaths from heart attacks and kidney failure. Life expectancy has improved with better medical care: the life expectancy of a child diagnosed with diabetes in the twenty-first century is longer than ever previously possible and may be nearly as good as that of a child who does not have diabetes. We also know that longevity is greatest in people who make regular visits to their doctor or practice nurse and who keep their diabetes under strict control. People who only have sporadic, infrequent supervision of their diabetes and those with poor control are more likely to die prematurely. Cigarette smokers are at particularly high risk. This is why we emphasise the importance of good control throughout this book.

My diabetes specialist has said that it does not follow that badly controlled people get all the side effects and ill health in later life and the reverse may often be true. Is this really so?

There is an element of truth in this but the word 'often' should be replaced by 'very occasionally'. Well controlled people are much less likely to become ill and develop side effects, whereas people who have unstable and unbalanced diabetes frequently develop ill health and side effects in later life. This has been confirmed by the results of the Diabetes Control and Complications Trial (DCCT) in the USA – there is more information about these trials in the section *Why monitor?* in Chapter 4.

I have had diabetes for the past ten years and have recently developed an unsightly skin condition on my shins. I was referred to a skin specialist who told me that it was related to my diabetes and would be very difficult to cure. What is it and why does it occur?

This is necrobiosis (Necrobiosis lipoidica diabeticorum) – a strange non-infectious but unsightly condition that usually occurs on the shins, but may occasionally appear elsewhere. Although it is associated with Type 1 diabetes and can develop at any time after diagnosis, on very rare occasions necrobosis may appear before diabetes itself, in which case it can be more difficult to diagnose. Nobody knows much about what causes it and treatment can be very disappointing, but achieving good control of diabetes may help. Local steroid injections and freezing with liquid nitrogen (cryotherapy) have been tried without much success. With time, the red raised patches quieten down and usually leave transparent scars. Diabetes UK have a necrobiosis network; this enables people with the condition to get in touch with others. You can contact the Diabetes UK Careline for more information. We know of one case where necrobiosis cleared up when the person stopped smoking.

EYES

I had a tendency towards short-sightedness before being diagnosed as having diabetes. Is this likely to increase my chances of developing eye complications later on?

Short-sightedness does not make the slightest difference to the risk of developing diabetic eye complications – in fact it has been said that those with severe short-sightedness may actually be less, rather than more, prone to retinopathy.

Vision may vary with changes in diabetes control. Large fluctuations in blood glucose levels can temporarily alter the shape of the lens in the eye and this alters its focusing capacity. It is not uncommon for people with consistently high blood glucose levels to have difficulty with distance vision. Once diabetes is controlled and the blood glucose returns to more normal levels, vision changes again, sometimes causing difficulty with near vision and therefore with reading.

These changes in vision are most likely to occur at the time diabetes is diagnosed and can be frightening, if the reason is not understood. After three or four weeks of good diabetic control, vision always returns to the prediabetes state. We always advise people with newly-diagnosed diabetes not to change their glasses until their blood glucose has been stable for about four weeks.

As someone with diabetes, I know I should have my eyes checked, but how often should this be?

Once a year should be enough if your diabetes is well controlled, your vision normal and you have no signs of complications. Diabetes can cause changes at the back of the eye (retinopathy). In the early stages, these changes do not affect vision but it is important to detect them as soon as possible so that treatment can be given to keep your vision normal. Nowadays, screening for retinopathy is usually carried out by digital photography and the Diabetes NSF states that this should be available to every person with diabetes.

I have just been found to have diabetes and have noticed that my glasses are not strong enough. I have been advised not change them – why is this?

When the glucose concentration is high, the eyes are unable to focus properly. This is only a temporary effect, and your vision will return to normal once the glucose has been brought under control. You should wait until your diabetes has been controlled for at least a month before going back to the optician.

Who is the best person to check my eyes once a year?

In the past, eye checks have been done in various ways but the Diabetes NSF recommends that every person with diabetes should be offered an annual eye check in the form of digital retinal photography (see next question on eye photography).

I have been sent an appointment for eye photographs. What will this involve?

There are two parts to the examination. The first is to test visual acuity, which measures your ability to read the letters on a chart. The second is to have the back of your eyes photographed. You will need drops in your eyes beforehand to enlarge the pupils in order to obtain good quality photographs. The drops may cause blurred vision for up to three hours afterwards and you should not drive until your vision has returned to normal. If it is a very bright day, you may suffer from glare while your pupils are dilated and sunglasses will prevent this. Each eye will be photographed once or twice using a flash camera. You may see some bright colours for a few seconds after the flash but these will go very quickly. If abnormalities are seen on the photographs, you will be referred to an eye specialist.

Last time I was having my eyes checked from the chart, the nurse made me look through a small pinhole. Why was this?

The pinhole acts as a universal correcting lens. If your vision improves when looking through the pinhole, it suggests that you may be helped by spectacles.

Why does diabetes affect the eyes?

A simple question but one that is difficult to answer. Current research indicates strongly that it is the excess glucose in the bloodstream that directly damages the eyes, mainly by affecting the lining of the small blood vessels that carry blood to the retina. The damage to these vessels seems to be directly related to how high the blood glucose is and how long it has been raised.

I have had diabetes for 20 years and seem to be quite well. Following my last eye photograph, I had a letter to say that I had some mild diabetic changes and would be referred to an eye specialist. Am I about to go blind?

There is no need for alarm. It would be surprising if there were no changes in your eyes after 20 years of diabetes. It is important that you see an eye specialist at an early stage so that if treatment is required, it can be given before your vision is affected.

I have been diagnosed with retinopathy. Can you explain more about this?

Retinopathy is a condition affecting the back of the eye (the retina). It may occur in people with long-standing diabetes, particularly those in whom control has not been very good. There is a gradual change in the blood vessels (arteries and veins) at the back of the eye which can lead to deterioration in vision. This may be due either to deposits in a vital area at the back of the eye or to bleeding into the eye from abnormal blood vessels.

Retinopathy may be diagnosed by examination of the eye with an ophthalmoscope or by retinal photography. It can usually be detected long before it leads to any disturbance in vision. Laser treatment at this stage usually stops further deterioration.

*On a recent TV programme it was stated that people with
diabetes over 40 years of age were likely to become blind.
This has horrified me because my 9-year-old son has diabetes
and unfortunately some of his school friends have told him
about the programme. What can I say to reassure him?*

It is almost inevitable that by the time someone has had diabetes for 20 years there will be some changes in the eyes (retinopathy). However, these are usually very minor and do not affect vision. Only a very small proportion of people actually go blind, probably no more than 7% of those who have had diabetes for 30 years or more. This figure is likely to reduce further over the next few years because the national retinopathy screening progamme has been set up to detect retinopathy at an early stage, when treatment can prevent damage to vision. We have known for 30 years that laser treatment is effective in treating diabetic retinopathy but sadly, some people do not realise they have a problem with their eyes until irreversible damage has been done. The retinal screening programme offers annual retinal photographs to everyone with diabetes over the age of 12 years so your son will soon be eligible for this. It is also worth explaining to your son that people with well controlled diabetes are much less likely to develop retinopathy than those with poor control.

*Can I wear contact lenses and if so would you recommend hard
or soft ones?*

The fact that you have diabetes should not interfere with your use of contact lenses or influence the sort of lens that you are given. The best person to advise you would be an ophthalmologist or qualified optician specialising in prescribing and fitting contact lenses. It would be sensible to let him or her know that you have diabetes and you must follow the advice given, particularly to prevent infection – but this applies to everyone, with or without diabetes.

I get flashes of light and specks across my vision. Are they symptoms of serious eye trouble?

Although people with diabetes do get eye trouble, this does not normally cause flashing lights or specks across the vision. You should discuss it with your own doctor who will want to examine your eyes in case there is any problem.

My father has diabetes and was recently told he had cataracts. Is this connected with his diabetes?

Cataracts occur in older people whether or not they have diabetes. However, they tend to occur at an earlier age in people with diabetes. The ageing process affects the substance that makes up the lens of the eye causing it to wrinkle and become less transparent than normal. Eventually it becomes so opaque that it becomes difficult to see properly through it. Your father's doctor should arrange for him to see an eye specialist.

My daughter aged 16 has just developed diabetes and her eyesight has deteriorated very rapidly. The doctor says she has cataracts but I thought that cataracts only occurred in old people. Can you explain what has happened?

There is a very rare form of cataract that can occur in childhood usually associated with very badly controlled diabetes. This is known as a 'snowstorm' cataract because of its characteristic appearance seen through an ophthalmoscope. This type of cataract can come on very rapidly and can be frightening if you do not know what has caused the poor vision. The cataract will need to be removed but there is no reason why your daughter should not have normal vision once this has been done.

The last time I was tested at the clinic, I was told that I had developed microaneurysms. What on earth are these?

Microaneurysms are little balloon-like swellings or dilatations in the very small blood vessels (capillaries) supplying the retina at the back of the eye. They are one of the earliest signs that the high blood glucose levels seen in poorly controlled diabetes have damaged the lining to these capillaries. They do not interfere with vision, but give an early warning that retinopathy has begun to develop. There is evidence to show that these can get better with the introduction of perfect control (target HbA_{1c} less than 7%) whereas, at later stages of diabetic retinopathy, reversal is not usually possible. Anyone who has microaneurysms must have regular eye checks, so that any serious developments are detected at an early stage.

I shall be going to have laser treatment soon on my eyes. What will this involve?

Laser treatment uses a narrow beam of intense light to cause very small burns on the retina at the back of the eye. It is used in the treatment of many eye conditions including diabetic retinopathy. The laser is directed at parts of the retina not used for detailed vision, sparing the important areas required for reading, etc. This form of treatment arrests or delays the progress of retinopathy, provided that it is given in adequate amounts at an early stage before useful vision is lost. It is sometimes necessary to give small doses of laser treatment intermittently over many years, although occasionally it can all be dealt with over a relatively short period. Although this treatment sounds quite alarming, it is not usually painful though it may cause minor discomfort.

My doctor used the term 'photocoagulation' the other day. Is this the same as laser treatment? Will it damage my eyes at all?

Photocoagulation is indeed treatment of retinopathy by lasers. It is uncommon for the treatment to damage the eyes, but strictly speaking it is possible. Occasionally the scar produced by photocoagulation can spread and involve vital parts of the retina so that vision is affected. The vast majority of people who have laser therapy do not notice any change in their vision. People who need repeated laser treatment may notice that their night vision is poor or that their field of vision is reduced. Photocoagulation can also very rarely result in rupture of a blood vessel, which causes bleeding. After a great deal of photocoagulation there is a slight risk of damage to the lens causing a type of cataract. Although this may sound rather worrying, there is very strong evidence to show that if you have serious retinopathy, laser treatment is the best way to preserve vision and the risk of damage as a result of the laser treatment is far less than the risk to your sight if the retinopathy is left untreated. It is important to realise that laser treatment cannot reverse any damage that has already occurred but it can prevent further deterioration.

I have glaucoma. Is this related to diabetes?

Possibly. Although glaucoma can occur quite commonly in people who do not have diabetes, there is a slightly increased risk in those who do. This is usually confined to those who have advanced diabetic eye problems (proliferative retinopathy).

Very occasionally the eye drops used to enlarge the pupil can precipitate an attack of glaucoma (increased pressure inside the eye). The signs of this are pain in the affected eye together with blurring of vision which may come on some hours after the drops have been put in. Should this occur you must seek urgent medical advice either from your own doctor or from the accident and emergency department of your local hospital. It is reversible with rapid treatment but can cause serious damage if ignored.

Every time I receive my copy of Balance, Diabetes UK's magazine, I have the impression that the print gets smaller. Is this true or is there something wrong with my eyes?

Eyesight tends to deteriorate with age, whether or not someone has diabetes. First you should visit your optician and have your eyesight checked to see whether it can be improved with glasses, as this may be all that is required. You should mention the fact that you have diabetes to your optician.

My eyesight has become very poor and my optician says it cannot be improved. I have increasing difficulty in reading. Is there any help available?

For people with eye problems severe enough to prevent reading, there are ways of helping. *Balance*, for example, is available to members of Diabetes UK as a cassette recording and this service is free of charge although, to satisfy Post Office regulations, you have to have a certificate of blindness before the cassette can be sent to you.

Public libraries can also help – most carry a wide selection of books in large type and also lend books on cassette and CD. Some larger libraries now have Kurtzweil machines, which can translate printed material into speech so that, in effect, they can read to you, although the 'voice' sounds a bit mechanical. This can be useful for any confidential material that you might not want another person to read to you. Libraries usually have these machines in rooms on their own so, once you have been shown how to use them, you can be quite private.

The Royal National Institute for the Blind also has an excellent talking book service. *Diabetes: Answers at your fingertips* is available as a talking book from the RNIB.

FEET, PODIATRY AND FOOTWEAR

I have just developed diabetes and have been warned that I am much more likely to get into trouble with my feet and need to take great care of them – what does this mean?

Diabetes can damage the nerves in the feet, reducing sensation and increasing the risk of injury and ulceration. If you keep your diabetes well controlled, have no loss of sensation and good circulation to your feet, you are no more at risk than a person without diabetes. If you do have nerve damage or poor circulation, you must protect your feet by taking the following precautions:

- inspecting your feet daily;

- keeping your toenails properly trimmed;

- avoiding badly fitting shoes.

When you have diabetes you should have access to the local registered podiatrist, who will check your feet and advise you, free of charge, on any questions that you may have.

I have had diabetes for ten years and as far as I can see it is quite under control and I am told that I am free from complications, but I cannot help worrying about the possibility of developing gangrene in the feet – can you tell me what it is and what causes it?

Gangrene results from tissue death. It can occur in any part of the body but most commonly affects the toes and fingers. Gangrene can occur in anyone with poor circulation and people with diabetes develop it only if they have a serious lack of blood supply to their feet. It can also be caused by smoking, which is the main cause of clogged-up blood vessels, and the combination of smoking and diabetes more than doubles the risk of gangrene.

There is another form of gangrene, which is caused by infection and is more common in people with diabetes. This usually affects the feet of people who have reduced sensation because of diabetic neuropathy (see the introduction to this chapter) and can occur even in the presence of a good blood supply. Any infected break in the skin of your feet must be taken seriously and treated promptly. If you are worried about anything to do with your feet, you should consult your doctor or podiatrist immediately. If the infection persists, ask to be referred to your local Diabetic Foot Team.

As someone with diabetes, do I have to take any special precautions when cutting my toenails?

It is important for everyone to cut their toenails to follow the shape of the end of the toe, and not cut deep into the corners. Your toenails should not be cut too short, and you should not use any sharp instrument to clean down the sides of the nails. All this is to avoid the possibility of ingrowing toenails. If you have problems cutting your toenails consult your registered podiatrist.

I have a thick callus on the top of one of my toes – can I use a corn plaster on this?

No, do not use any corn remedies on your feet. They often contain an acid which softens the skin and increases the risk of an infection. Consult a registered podiatrist to have it treated. Contacts can be found on the websites for the Society of Chiropodists and Podiatrists and the Health Professions Council. As you have diabetes you should have access to a registered podiatrist who will treat you free of charge.

My son has picked up athlete's foot. He has diabetes treated with insulin – do I have to take any special precautions about using the powder and cream given to me by my doctor?

No. Athlete's foot is very common and is due to a fungal infection, which should respond quickly to treatment with the appropriate antifungal preparation; this can be bought without prescription. Do not forget the usual precautions of making sure he keeps his feet clean, dries them carefully and changes his socks daily. Try to encourage him not to wear the same footwear every day.

Will I get bunions because I have diabetes?

No. Bunions are no more common in people who have diabetes than in those who do not.

I have had diabetes for 25 years and I have been warned that the sensation in my feet is not normal. I am troubled with an ingrowing toenail on my big toe, which often gets red but does not hurt – what should I do?

You should urgently seek help and advice in case it is infected. If so, you are at risk of the infection spreading without you being aware of it, because it would hurt less than in someone with normal sensation. This is potentially a serious situation, so see your doctor or podiatrist straight away.

I am 67 and have had diabetes for 15 years. As far as I can tell my feet are quite healthy but, as my vision is not very good, I find it difficult to inspect my feet properly – what can I do about it?

Do you have a friend or relative who could look at your feet regularly and trim your nails? If this is not possible, then the sensible thing to do would be to see a podiatrist regularly. Ask your GP or diabetes clinic about local arrangements for seeing a registered podiatrist.

MORECAMBE BAY HOSPITALS NHS TRUST

Feet Facts

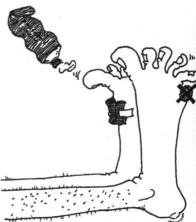

✱ Minor cuts or abrasions can be covered with sterile gauze after use of a mild antiseptic cream.

✱ Avoid using corn plasters – they contain acids which can cause problems.

✱ Don't prick blisters, instead treat as for a minor abrasion.

✱ Corns, calluses or ingrowing toenails must always be treated by your chiropodist.

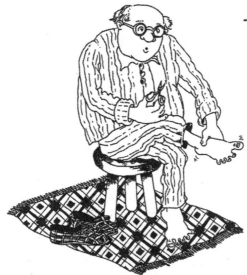

✱ When your toenails need cutting, always do this after bathing.

✱ Cut the nail edge following the shape of the end of the toe.

✱ Don't cut the corners of your toenails back into the nail grooves.

✱ Avoid using a sharp instrument to clean the free nail edge or the nail grooves.

Figure 9.1 Foot care information

* If your skin is too dry, apply a small amount of emollient cream (e.g. E45).

* Check and bathe your feet every day, then pat dry gently, particularly between the toes.

* If your skin is moist, dab gently with surgical spirit and then dust lightly with talcum powder.

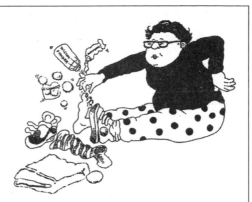

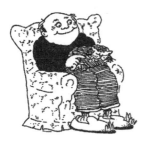

* Remove hot water bottles before getting into bed, and switch off your electric blanket.

* If thick woollen bed-socks are worn, they must be loose fitting.

* Be careful not to sit too close to radiators or fires.

* Choose shoes which provide good support. They must be broad, long and deep enough. Check that you can wriggle all your toes.

* Shoes should have a fastening.

* Check shoes daily for any small objects, such as hairpins, stones or buttons.

* If socks have ridges or seams, wear them inside out. Loose fitting ones are best.

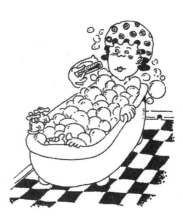

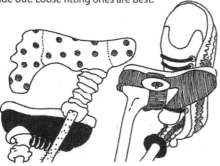

* Avoid very hot baths.

* Always dry your feet carefully after bathing.

Do I have to pay for chiropody?

Most hospital diabetes departments provide a chiropody (podia-try) service free of charge. Outside the hospital service, chiropody under the NHS is based on locally agreed priority groups. Most districts consider people with diabetes as a priority group and do offer free chiropody. You should check locally before obtaining treatment. If you are seeing a podiatrist privately, make sure that he or she is registered (see question on corn plasters, above, for details).

How can I tell whether diabetes is affecting my feet?

Diabetes may affect the feet in two major ways. The first is caused by reduced blood supply from arterial thickening, sometimes called 'hardening of the arteries' or atherosclerosis. This leads to poor circulation with cold feet, even in warm weather, and cramps in the calf when you are walking (intermittent claudication). Poor circulation is not confined to people with diabetes and becomes increasingly common with age, particularly in people who smoke. The combination of diabetes and smoking is particularly harmful and in severe cases this can progress to gangrene.

The second way that diabetes can affect the feet is through damage to the nerves (neuropathy), which reduces the feeling of pain and awareness of extremes of temperature. When your feet are insensitive, it is easy to damage them without realising it, for example by wearing poorly fitting footwear. Neuropathy can be quite difficult to detect unless the feet are examined by an expert. Once a year, one of the health professionals helping you to manage your diabetes should examine your feet for signs of reduced blood supply or nerve damage. They should tell you if there is evidence that diabetes is affecting your feet.

The danger is that any minor damage to the foot, whether from a cut or abrasion or a badly fitting shoe, will not cause the usual painful reaction, so that damage can result from continued injury or from infection. It is important that you know whether the sensation in your feet is normal or reduced. Make sure that you ask your doctor or nurse about this at your next review.

My daughter has diabetes and often walks barefoot around the house. Should I discourage her from doing this?

It is well known that people with diabetes are prone to problems with their feet which are, for the most part, due to carelessness and can be avoided. The usual reason these problems occur is that, with increasing duration of diabetes, sensation in the feet tends to be reduced. Most people are unaware of this, and so the danger is that damage to the feet may be the first indication of the problem. By then it could be too late!

However, the dangers to the feet of children and teenagers with diabetes are really very slight and there is no reason to discourage your daughter from walking about barefoot.

What special care should I take of my feet during the winter?

In older people with diabetes, the blood supply to the feet may not be very good and this will make their feet more vulnerable to damage by severe cold. As winter is cold and wet, we tend to wear warmer clothing, and previously comfortable shoes may become unpleasantly tight when worn with thick woolly socks or stockings. This may reduce the circulation to the feet and can numb the sensation completely, leading to damage. All these effects will be made worse if your feet become wet.

Make sure your shoes are comfortable, fit well, and allow room for you to wear an adequately thick pair of socks, preferably made of wool or other absorbent material. Use weather-proof shoes, over-shoes or boots if you are going to be out for any length of time in the rain or snow, and dry your feet carefully if they get wet. Do not put your cold – and slightly numb – feet straight onto a hot-water bottle or near a hot fire because you may find that, when the feeling comes back, the heat is excessive and chilblains may occur. Feet also need protection during the summer as wearing open sandals can cause problems from possible damage by sharp stones, etc.

How can I give continual protection to my feet?

It is extremely difficult. If the sensation in your feet is normal, then generally you have very little need to worry but, if there is even slight numbness of your feet, you should check them daily and ask someone else to look at the areas that you have difficulty seeing. (If there is no one to ask you could try using a mirror to look at the soles of your feet.) You are looking for signs mentioned in the **Foot Care Rules** (Figure 9.2). If your circulation is poor, try hard to keep your feet warm and well protected.

I have suffered from foot ulcers for many years and would be grateful if you could suggest something to help my problem.

You should not attempt to treat these yourself. Seek medical advice and expert podiatry, usually provided by your local Diabetic Foot Team. Foot ulcers in people with diabetes are usually caused by reduced sensation in the feet (neuropathy) and you should have your feet examined by your specialist to find out whether this is the case. If so, you need to attend for regular podiatry and learn all the ways of avoiding trouble when sensation is reduced. You may need special shoes made by a shoe fitter (an orthotist), which your consultant or podiatrist can arrange. Another form of treatment for people with foot ulcers is to use a removeable plaster cast, such as is used to immobilise fractured bones. These can be made from a light plastic material called Scotchcast, which provides maximum protection to an ulcerated foot.

*I have so many other things to remember – can you give me a
simple list of rules for foot care?*

The **Foot Care Rules** (Figure 9.2) are aimed specifically at those
who have either poor blood supply (ischaemia) or nerve damage
(neuropathy). If you have poor eyesight then you should get somebody else with good eyesight to help you inspect and care for your
feet. The rules are shown in a more entertaining form in Figure 9.1.

I have a swollen foot – is this to do with my diabetes?

Swelling of both feet, especially towards the end of the day, is not
directly related to diabetes and there are a number of possible
causes, some of which may benefit from treatment. The best thing
would be to speak to your doctor about this.

Sometimes people with diabetes and reduced sensation in their
feet (neuropathy) can develop a swollen, painful foot which is warm
to the touch and can look like a sprained ankle. This uncommon
condition is called a Charcot foot and it is important to recognise and
treat it at an early stage. If left untreated the foot may change shape,
which will put it at increased risk of ulceration in the future. The
Charcot process may start as a result of a minor injury to the foot
and the diagnosis is often delayed because the changes are thought
to be due to a sprain. It is very important to see your GP or podiatrist
as soon as possible as if you have this condition you will need specialist treatment from the Diabetes Foot Team.

The treatment for a Charcot foot is to immobilise it in a cast – this
can be a traditional plaster cast or an aircast (sometimes called a
'Beckham Boot') to stop the foot changing shape. Sometimes tablets
normally used for osteoporosis (bisphosphonates) are prescribed to
strengthen the bones. It can take several months for a Charcot foot to
stabilise but if during this time you protect your foot from changing
shape, it will be worth the inconvenience.

Figure 9.2 Foot care rules

FOOT CARE RULES

DOs

- **Do** wash your feet daily with soap and warm water. Do not use hot water – check the temperature of the water with your elbow.
- **Do** dry your feet well with a soft towel; be especially gentle between your toes.
- **Do** apply a gentle skin cream, such as E45, if your skin is rough and dry.
- **Do** change your socks or stockings daily and keep them in good repair.
- **Do** wear well-fitting shoes. Make sure they are wider, deeper and longer than your foot with a good firm fastening that you have to undo to get your foot in and out. This will prevent your foot from moving inside the shoe.
- **Do** run your hand around the inside of your shoes each day before putting them on to check that there is nothing that will rub your feet.
- **Do** 'wear in' new shoes for short periods of time and check your feet afterwards to see if the shoe has rubbed or pinched your feet.
- **Do** cut your toenails to follow the shape of the end of your toes, not deep into the corners. This is easier after a bath as your toenails will soften in the warm water.
- **Do** check your feet daily and see your podiatrist or doctor about any problems.
- **Do** see a registered podiatrist if in any doubt about foot care.

DON'Ts

- **Do not** soak your feet.
- **Do not** put your feet on hot-water bottles or sit too close to a fire or radiator, and avoid extremes of cold and heat.

- **Do not** use corn paints or plasters or attempt to cut your own corns with knives or razors under any circumstances.
- **Do not** neglect even slight injuries to your feet.
- **Do not** walk barefoot.
- **Do not** let your feet get dry and cracked. Use E45 or hand lotion to keep the skin soft. Avoid putting moisturiser between the toes.
- **Do not** cut your toenails too short or dig down the sides of your nails.
- **Do not** smoke.

Seek advice immediately if you notice any of the following:

- Any colour change in your legs or feet;
- Any discharge from a break or crack in the skin, or from a corn or from beneath a toenail;
- Any swelling, throbbing or signs of inflammation (redness or heat) in any part of your foot.

First aid measures

- Minor injuries can be treated at home provided that professional help is sought if the injury does not improve quickly.
- Minor cuts and abrasions should be cleaned gently with cotton wool or gauze and warm salt water. A clean dressing should be lightly bandaged in place.
- If blisters occur, do not prick them. If they burst, dress as for minor cuts.
- Never use strong medicaments such as iodine.
- Never place adhesive strapping directly over a wound: always apply a dressing first.

KIDNEY DAMAGE

It's bad enough having diabetes. If I'm also at risk of kidney damage, what should I look for?

Diabetes may affect the kidneys in several ways, and the routine urine and blood tests that you have once a year, either at your doctor's surgery or at your diabetes clinic, can detect changes at an early stage, when it is possible for treatment to protect against further damage.

Large amounts of glucose in the urine put you at risk of infection that can spread from the bladder (cystitis) up to the kidneys (pyelonephritis). Sometimes long-standing kidney infections may cause very few symptoms and are only revealed by routine urine tests.

People with long-standing and poorly controlled diabetes are at risk of damage to the small blood vessels supplying the kidney, in the same way that the retina of the eye may be affected. This does not produce any symptoms but will be detected with a urine test carried out by your doctor or nurse. Most clinics now test for 'microalbuminuria', which as the name implies is a microscopic amount of albumin (protein) in the urine. This is a very useful test as it can detect very minor kidney damage, which will respond to treatment.

With more severe kidney disease, large amounts of albumin may be lost in the urine. This may make the urine froth and can lead to a build-up of fluid in the body, which in turn leads to swelling around the ankles (oedema). Over many years, these changes may progress to kidney failure. This is usually detected by blood tests and urine tests years before the symptoms develop.

I have developed kidney failure. Will it be possible to have dialysis or even a transplant although I have diabetes?

Yes. The majority of people who are unfortunate enough to get kidney failure are suitable for both forms of treatment.

Dialysis (or renal replacement therapy) is of two major types. The older type is haemodialysis where the blood is washed in a special machine three times a week. The more recent form of dialysis is known as CAPD (chronic ambulatory peritoneal dialysis) where fluid is washed in and out of the abdomen three or four times a day. The benefit of CAPD is that it can be carried out at home and does not need sophisticated machinery. People with diabetes seem to be very good at learning this method, which is simpler and cheaper than haemodialysis.

Transplantation is the aim of most dialysis programmes, but the supply of suitable kidneys is a limiting factor. The source of kidneys is either from people dying accidentally or from a family member who has agreed to give one of their kidneys to a relative with kidney failure. A normal person can manage perfectly well with one kidney without reducing their life expectancy provided the kidney does not get damaged. The donor will, of course, have to have an operation and will be slightly more vulnerable as a result because they will have only one kidney to rely on instead of two.

I was found to have protein (albumin) in my urine when I last attended the diabetes clinic – what does this mean?

If it was only a trace of protein, it may mean nothing, but you should have your urine checked again to make sure it is now clear. If the protein is still present, it suggests either that you could have an infection in the bladder or kidney (cystitis or pyelonephritis) or that you have developed a degree of diabetic kidney damage (nephropathy). There are many other causes of protein (albumin) in the urine and it may not be related to your diabetes. If the protein is always present in every urine specimen, this should be investigated, and you should ask to be kept informed of the results of the tests.

At my last clinic visit I was told that I had microalbuminuria.
What is this?

One of the effects diabetes can have on the kidney is to cause protein (albumin) to leak into the urine. At first this happens in microscopic amounts, but with time the albumin in the urine (albuminuria) increases and this can lead to fluid retention and ankle swelling. A very sensitive test has been developed to detect albumin at the microscopic stage (microalbuminuria) and your doctor or nurse should ask you to provide an early morning urine sample once a year so that you can be tested for microalbuminuria. The reason for screening for kidney damage at such an early stage is that if it is detected, microalbuminuria can be stabilised or even reversed by keeping the blood pressure absolutely normal and by treating you with a tablet known as an ACE inhibitor. For the same reason it is important to keep your diabetes as well controlled as possible.

At my last diabetes check my doctor told me that I had a
condition called microalbuminuria and that I needed to take a
blood pressure tablet to protect my kidneys, even though he says
my blood pressure is normal. I feel very well and don't like the
idea of taking tablets. Is this really necessary?

It is always difficult to accept the need to take treatment when you are feeling perfectly well and most people are reluctant to take tablets in these circumstances. However, there is good evidence that microalbuminuria can be halted, and can even be reversed, by treatment with an ACE inhibitor and your doctor is giving you good advice.

NERVE DAMAGE

There are a number of conditions that can affect the nervous system of someone with diabetes: diabetic neuritis, diabetic neuropathy, autoimmune neuropathy and diabetic amyotrophy. We discuss these below.

I have been on insulin for three years. Eighteen months ago I started to get pains in both legs and could barely walk. Despite treatment I am still suffering. Can you tell me what can be done to ease this pain?

There are many causes of leg pains, and only one is due specifically to diabetes. This is a particularly vicious form of nerve damage called neuritis, which causes singularly unpleasant pain, chiefly in the feet or thighs, or sometimes both. The pain is often described as pins and needles, or constant burning, and is often worse at night causing lack of sleep. Contact with clothes or bed-clothes is often acutely uncomfortable.

Fortunately this form of neuritis is rather uncommon and always disappears, although it may last for many months before subsiding. Sometimes good control of your diabetes will help to alleviate the symptoms and speed recovery. Relief can be obtained by simple painkillers, but there are also some drugs which were developed for other purposes which have been shown to be effective in relieving pain due to neuropathy. The first choice is the antidepressant amitriptyline. If this fails, gabapentin or pregabalin, which were first developed for epilepsy, should be tried. Sometimes sleeping tablets can help. As a general rule, painful neuropathy improves eventually but this can take some time.

*I have had diabetes for many years but my general health is
good and I am very stable. During the last year, however, I have
developed an extreme soreness on the soles of my feet whenever
pressure has been applied, such as when digging with a spade,
standing on ladders, walking on hard ground or stones, even
when applying the accelerator in the car. If I thump an object
with the palm of my hand, I suffer the same soreness. The pain
is extreme and sometimes lasts for a day or so. Could you tell me
if you have heard of this condition in other people and what is
the reason for it?*

These symptoms may be due to diabetic neuropathy, a condition of
damage to the nerves, which sometimes occurs in long-standing
diabetes. It affects the feet more often than other parts of the body
and may cause painful tingling or burning sensations in the feet,
although numbness is perhaps more common. Strict control of your
diabetes is important for the prevention and treatment of this complication – it can be made worse by moderate or high alcohol
consumption.

*I suffer from neuritis in my face. My GP says there is no
apparent reason for this but I wondered if it had anything to do
with my diabetes.*

Not necessarily, as there are a number of types of neuritis that
can affect the face, which have absolutely nothing to do with
diabetes. Examples include both shingles (*Herpes zoster*) and Bell's
palsy, although, of course, both these conditions can affect people
with diabetes.

There are forms of diabetic neuritis that do affect the face: one
form occasionally affects the muscles of the eye leading to double
vision, while another form can cause numbness and tingling. There
is also a very rare complication known as 'gustatory sweating' where
sweating breaks out across the head and scalp at the start of a meal.

I have recently been told that the tingling sensation in my fingers is due to carpal tunnel syndrome and not neuropathy as was first thought. Can you please explain the difference?

Carpal tunnel syndrome commonly occurs in people who do not have diabetes; the wrist compresses the nerve supplying the skin over the fingers, the palm of the hand and some of the muscles in the hand. Occasionally, injections of hydrocortisone or related steroids into the wrist will relieve it. Sometimes a small operation at the wrist to relieve the tension on the nerve may be required. This usually brings about a dramatic relief of any associated pain and a recovery of sensation and muscle strength with time.

Diabetic neuropathy more commonly affects the feet than the hands and is usually a painless loss of sensation starting with the tips of the toes or fingers and moving up the legs or arms. It is only occasionally painful and may be difficult to treat. It is due to generalised damage to the nerves, not to compression of any one nerve and is often described as 'glove and stocking' because of the areas it affects.

I have had diabetes for 27 years and have recently had a lot of trouble with diarrhoea. My doctor says it may be caused by diabetes. Could you explain why this should happen now and how it can be treated?

Diabetic diarrhoea is one of a number of problems which can be caused by autonomic neuropathy. This occurs when there is damage to the nerves supplying the 'automatic' bodily functions such as bowels, bladder and stomach. It is an uncommon condition, which can develop after many years of diabetes. For reasons which are not well understood, the symptoms may come and go and can affect different parts of the body at different times. In your case, the nerves that regulate the activity of your bowels have been affected. This is a distressing condition particularly as the diarrhoea often occurs at night. It may respond to a short course of antibiotics, which can be repeated if the diarrhoea returns. Standard diarrhoea treatments such as loperamide may be helpful. Irritable bowel syndrome can cause symptoms not unlike this – although it has nothing to do with diabetes. If you ever see blood or mucus in your stools, you should seek medical advice without delay.

I have had diabetes for more than 30 years and have had a lot of problems with vomiting recently. This has made my blood sugar levels rather unpredictable. Is there an explanation for this?

In people who have had diabetes for many years, vomiting can be caused by a condition called gastroparesis. This results from damage to the nerves supplying the stomach (autonomic neuropathy). It is not uncommon for people to vomit food eaten several hours earlier because the stomach becomes paralysed and floppy and the food does not move through the digestive system in the normal way. This can lead to unpredictable blood glucose levels because the food is absorbed slowly and erratically. If you suffer from this condition it may be a good idea to delay your insulin injection until after you have eaten and your blood glucose has started to rise. It may be helped by anti-vomiting tablets such as metoclopramide.

The calf muscle in one leg seems to be shrinking. There is no ache and no pain. Is this anything to do with diabetes? I have been taking insulin for 30 years.

You do not mention whether you have noticed any weakness in this leg. Occasionally, diabetic neuropathy can affect the nerves which supply the muscles, causing the muscle to become weak and shrink in size without any accompanying pain or discomfort. It sounds as if this may be your problem.

I have had diabetes for many years and have developed pain in my legs. My thighs in particular are very weak and wasted. I have been told that I have 'diabetic amyotrophy'. Will it get better?

Diabetic amyotrophy is a rare condition causing pain and weakness of one or both legs and is due to damage to nerves. It usually occurs when diabetes control is very poor, but occasionally affects people with only slight elevation of the blood glucose. Strict control of diabetes leads to its improvement but it may take up to two years or so for it to settle. The nerves affected are usually those supplying the thigh muscles, as in your case, which become wasted and weak.

HEART AND BLOOD VESSEL DISEASE

I have read that poor circulation in the feet is a problem for people with diabetes. Is there any way I can improve my circulation to avoid developing this?

Narrowing ('hardening') of the arteries is a normal part of growing older – and the arteries to the feet can be affected by this process, leading to poor circulation in the feet and legs. The causes of arterial disease are not very well understood, but we know that smoking and poor diabetes control make it worse. So if you have diabetes and smoke cigarettes, the risk of bad circulation increases greatly. The best advice is to stop smoking, control your blood glucose, and keep active – regular exercise will encourage the circulation to improve. Your doctor should be treating you with a statin to lower your cholesterol. If you are unfortunate enough to develop circulation problems your GP can refer you to a vascular surgeon to see if the arteries can be unblocked. This can sometimes be done by inserting a tube with a small balloon into the artery (angioplasty) or alternatively by an operation to bypass the blockage.

I am worried that I might develop heart problems. I am already being treated for high blood pressure. Is heart disease likely?

Heart disease is up to five times more common in people with diabetes and goes hand in hand with high blood pressure and raised cholesterol. These risk factors are important causes of premature death in people with diabetes. We know that controlling blood pressure, cholesterol and blood glucose reduces the chances of developing heart disease and there are now recommended targets for blood pressure, cholesterol and blood glucose, which your GP or practice nurse should be helping you to achieve.

These targets are:

- HbA_{1c}: 6.5–7.5%;

- Cholesterol (total): less than 4.0; LDL less than 2.0 mmol/L;

- Blood pressure: less than 140/80 unless you have micro-albuminuria or proteinuria, when it should be less than 135/75.

I am 26 and have Type 1 diabetes. I am already taking treatment for blood pressure because I have a small amount of protein in the urine and now my doctor has recommended that I take a tablet to lower my cholesterol. Is this really necessary at my age?

It is always difficult to know what advice to give to young people with diabetes because most of the research studies which have shown benefit from lowering cholesterol have only included people over the age of 40. Some doctors would advise cholesterol-lowering tablets for anyone with diabetes over the age of 18 but this may seem rather extreme. There is, however, good evidence that the risk of heart trouble is greater if you already have complications of diabetes such as protein in the urine. Most specialists would recommend a cholesterol-lowering tablet in your situation.

Young women with diabetes must be very careful to avoid pregnancy while taking tablets for cholesterol or blood pressure as they can harm the developing baby. Anyone planning a pregnancy should stop their medication before trying to conceive as damage can occur before you know you are pregnant. Stopping the tablets for a few months will not cause any long-term problems.

Recently I have had some pain in my chest. My doctor says it could be angina and wants me to see a heart specialist for tests. What is angina and what will these tests involve?

Angina is a heart pain which occurs when the blood supply to the heart is insufficient because of narrowing of the coronary arteries. It is usually brought on by exercise, because that is when the heart needs most blood, but if the narrowing of the arteries is very severe, it may happen at rest. If one of the arteries becomes completely blocked, this leads to a heart attack. It is sometimes possible to improve the coronary circulation, either by inserting a small tube called a stent or by an operation to bypass the blockage.

The heart specialist may want to carry out various tests which may include asking you to walk on a treadmill while recording your heart tracing. He or she may also want to inject dye into the coronary arteries to identify the site of the blockage. This is normally done by inserting a tube into your groin area using a local anaesthetic. If it is not possible to correct the blockage, there are a number of treatments available which can widen the coronary arteries and prevent blood clots.

I am in my early twenties, but haven't had good diabetes control for a couple of years. Will this affect my arteries in later life?

It is unlikely to have much effect at your age but if you continue to have poor control over the next few years, you are likely to build up trouble for the future. Our arteries get more rigid and more clogged up as we get older and this process can be aggravated by periods of poor diabetes control and by smoking.

I have had diabetes for 40 years and unfortunately my left leg had to be amputated because I developed gangrene. I now get a lot of pain in my right foot and calf. Could too much insulin be the cause of this pain?

It sounds as if the blood supply to your leg is insufficient and that this is the cause of the pain in your right foot and calf. As you know, this is the reason you developed gangrene in your left leg and you must be very worried about your right leg. You should tell your doctor about the pain as you may need to be referred to a vascular surgeon to see if anything can be done to improve the blood supply to your foot (see first question in this section).

There are a number of things you can do to help protect your remaining leg and these include:

- stopping smoking (if you smoke);
- keeping diabetes, blood pressure and cholesterol under very good control;
- maintaining close contact with a podiatrist who has a special interest in diabetes.

If you notice any sign of increased pain or change in colour, you should seek medical advice immediately.

My husband had a heart attack last year. Nine months later he had part of his leg amputated. We have been told that he could have further problems but have been given no advice. Please give us some information on what we should do to try and avoid this.

It sounds as though your husband has generalised arterial disease (arteriosclerosis) affecting the blood vessels to the heart and to the leg. There are a number of things which you and he can do that may be of help in preventing further trouble.

- If he smokes, he should stop straight away.

- He should take a statin to reduce cholesterol; the target is less than 4 mmol/L.

- He should keep his diabetes and blood pressure as well controlled as possible. The target is HbA$_{1c}$ 6.5–7.5% and blood pressure less than 140/80.

- He should keep his remaining foot and leg warm and make sure that he has expert foot care from a podiatrist. If you see any signs of damage to his foot or any discoloration seek medical advice immediately.

BLOOD PRESSURE

I have been told that my blood pressure is raised as a result of diabetic kidney problems and, because of this, it is very important that I take tablets to lower it – why is this?

There is good evidence to show that lowering the blood pressure to normal protects the kidneys from further damage. We also know that controlling blood pressure reduces the risk of heart disease and stroke. Studies in Germany and the UK have shown that blood pressure can be reduced significantly if people participate actively by self-monitoring of blood pressure. In these studies, participants were provided with a blood pressure monitor and given information about reducing high blood pressure; this included non-drug remedies, such as reducing salt, increasing fruit and vegetable intake and exercising. They were taught how to use an individual flow chart so they could make their own decisions about medication. The British Hypertension Society (address in Appendix 2) provides advice on how to select a reliable monitor, and if you think that you may benefit from self-monitoring of blood pressure, you should discuss this with your doctor or nurse.

I have been suffering from dizzy spells recently and on a couple of occasions I have fainted after standing up suddenly. My doctor says that this may be due to low blood pressure as a result of diabetes but I thought that diabetes caused high blood pressure. Can you explain?

Dizziness on standing up, sometimes known as postural hypotension, can be caused by autonomic neuropathy, when damage to the nerves controlling the blood pressure prevents the body from adjusting to changes in posture. This can lead to a rapid fall in blood pressure, most noticeable when you are standing up. The problem is made worse by poor control of diabetes, which can lead to dehydration. You should try to make sure that your diabetes is well controlled and if the problem persists you should see your GP. A tablet called fludrocortisone, which leads to fluid retention, can often help this condition.

THE MIND

My 68-year-old mother has had diabetes for 44 years. In the past few years her mental state has deteriorated considerably and she has difficulty looking after herself. Is this common for someone who has been on insulin for so long?

Your mother's memory loss may be due either to Alzheimer's disease, brain damage due to hardening of the arteries (arteriosclerosis) or possibly to repeated hypos over more than 40 years. As you know, both memory loss and diabetes are found in older people so the two conditions may occur together. Alzheimer's disease may be slightly more common in people with diabetes but there is no clear explanation for this. Arteriosclerosis is a complication of diabetes, which may affect the arteries to the brain as well as the heart or legs. Controlling blood pressure, cholesterol and blood glucose will reduce this risk. Finally it seems that people on insulin, whose blood glucose is usually below normal with repeated hypos over 30 or 40 years, may eventually develop memory loss.

I had a brain haemorrhage 18 months ago and I have had diabetes since childhood. Am I more likely to get complications from diabetes?

Brain haemorrhages and strokes are more common in people with diabetes, particularly if blood pressure levels are high. Since you have already had a stroke, you may be more at risk of other circulatory problems. This makes it particularly important that the usual risk factors (blood pressure, cholesterol and blood glucose) are kept under tight control. There is recent evidence that taking a high dose of a statin to reduce the cholesterol to very low levels has an additional benefit in lowering the risk of further stroke. Your doctor and nurse will be keen to help you with this.

I have been very depressed since my diagnosis. Are people with diabetes more prone to depression?

Having to deal with the many demands of diabetes is bound to cause you to feel gloomy at times and this seems to be most likely when it hits home that you have diabetes for life with no chance of a holiday from it. When large populations have been studied, depression in diabetes is found to be about twice as common as in people without diabetes.

If your depression does not clear, you must tell your GP about it. Just because you have diabetes, it does not mean that your depression should not be addressed and treated in the normal way. Depression is dealt with elsewhere in this book – see p. 150.

I have read that hypos can cause brain damage – is this true?

It is possible for a severe hypo leading to unconsciousness for hours or days to cause permanent brain damage. However, this cannot result from 'normal' hypos that occur in the course of living with diabetes and insulin. In practice, brain damage only occurs when someone on insulin takes a deliberate overdose as a suicide attempt. The tragic consequence of a failed attempt on one's life by insulin overdose is that it can lead to severe brain damage and a life of complete dependence on others.

There is also a suspicion that people who have repeated hypos for 20 or 30 years may have a form of memory loss late in life. However, this is only conjecture and has never been proved.

10 | Research and the future

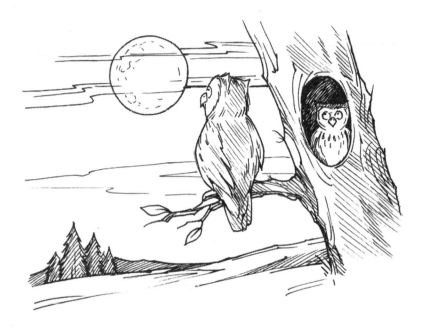

New developments and improvements in existing treatments can occur only through research; therefore research is vital to every person with diabetes. In the UK, Diabetes UK spends large sums (approximately £5 million each year) on research into diabetes. Voluntary groups of Diabetes UK put a lot of energy into fundraising for the benefit of everyone with diabetes. There is always a need for more money because there are many good research ideas which are not funded. Other grant-giving bodies, such as the Medical Research Council and the Wellcome Trust contribute large sums to diabetes research. At the time of writing, it costs about £30,000 to support a relatively junior research worker for just one year.

The most inspiring research project in diabetes was the discovery of insulin itself in 1921, when a doctor and a medical student (Banting and Best) worked together during a few summer months to produce a life-saving treatment. There have been many important but less dramatic discoveries since then, each in some way contributing to our understanding of diabetes and many improving the available treatment.

Look at the Diabetes UK website for details of Diabetes UK research activities (see Appendix 2).

SEARCHING FOR CAUSES AND CURES

Do you think that diabetes will ever be cured?

Ever since a life-saving treatment for diabetes became available in 1922, there has been a constant search for a cure, which would relieve people of the burden of living with this condition. Great advances have been made in our understanding of the causes of Type 1 and Type 2 diabetes and at times it has looked as if a cure was just around the corner. Sadly these were false dawns but a huge amount of research effort continues to be devoted to trying to find a cure.

Will it ever be possible to prevent diabetes with a vaccine?

There is some evidence to suggest that certain virus infections can cause diabetes but we are not clear how often this happens: it is probably very infrequently. If we were able to identify a virus, it might be possible to produce a vaccine which could be given to children in the same way as other childhood vaccines. At present this possibility seems rather remote.

GENETICS

I have heard that it may be possible to test members of families at high risk of diabetes to predict who may go on to get diabetes in the future. How is this done and will it be possible to treat those at risk to prevent diabetes from developing?

A lot of research work has been carried out in families in whom two or three members have Type 1 diabetes. This has shown that some of the so-called HLA tissue antigens are associated with a high frequency of diabetes and that people whose blood contains antibodies to the insulin-producing cells of the pancreas are likely to develop diabetes within a few years. These genetic and antibody markers can be detected in a blood sample and it is thus possible to identify family members at risk. The next step is to try to stop the process whereby insulin-secreting cells are destroyed, thereby preventing diabetes. So far no one has managed to find a way of doing this (see following questions).

Is it true that studying families who have several members with diabetes can help find a cure for the condition?

Family studies are very important in helping to understand the inheritance of diabetes. In some families there is a clear association between a certain genetic make-up and the development of diabetes. Those members who have not yet developed diabetes may have the 'markers' (see previous question), indicating that they are at increased risk.

Is it possible to prevent diabetes in people with a high risk of developing Type 1 diabetes?

As described in previous answers, it is known that Type 1 diabetes develops because the islet cells in the pancreas which produce insulin are damaged by antibodies and once a critical number have been destroyed, the blood glucose rises and diabetes ensues. It is possible to identify close relatives of children with Type 1 diabetes in whom this process of islet cell destruction has begun. Several methods have been tried to halt the destruction in the hope of preventing diabetes, some of which are mentioned here.

- **Insulin as prevention** This project started in 1994 and relatives who had high levels of islet cell antibodies were entered into the study. Half the people with diabetes were asked to take a small dose of long-acting insulin twice a day for up to 5 years; the rest were controls who were simply observed. Unfortunately all those insulin injections had no effect in reducing the risk of diabetes.

- **Ciclosporin** This immune suppressant drug was given to young people at risk of diabetes identified by antibody and genetic markers. Those taking the drug had a slower progression to diabetes for as long as they took it. However, there were worries about long-term immune suppression in young people and the treatment was stopped after 12 months. As soon as ciclosporin was stopped the progression to diabetes took off again.

- **Nicotinamide** There was some evidence from New Zealand that the vitamin nicotinamide slowed down the development of diabetes in young people. A large study was set up in the UK whereby children at risk were identified in the usual way. Half the children were asked to take tablets of nicotinamide every day for five years and the control group took placebo (dummy) tablets. After five years of treatment with nicotinamide, the number of people with diabetes was the same in both groups. Thus nicotinamide was not effective in preventing diabetes in young people at risk.

- **Monoclonal antibodies** In this study, artificial antibodies were manufactured against CD3 lymphocytes which play a part in the process of islet cell destruction. These antibodies were given over six consecutive days to people who had the warning signs of diabetes in their blood. Eighteen months after treatment, the group who had received the antibody needed 60% less insulin and had better control of their diabetes than the comparison group.

TRANSPLANTATION

I should like to volunteer to have a pancreas transplant. Is there someone I must apply to? How successful have these operations been?

Pancreatic transplantation is still in the experimental stages and you are unlikely to find anyone who will accept you as a volunteer. Technically, pancreatic transplants are even more difficult than liver, kidney or heart transplants. The pancreas is very delicate but also produces digestive juices, which digest the pancreas itself if it is damaged while being removed from the donor and placed in the recipient. The duct or tube through which these juices pass is narrow, and has to be joined up to the intestines in an intricate way so that the enzymes do not leak. Even if the procedure is a technical success, the body will still reject the transplant unless powerful drugs are given to suppress the immune system. Some of these (particularly steroids) tend to cause diabetes or make existing diabetes worse. Some UK transplant centres will offer people with diabetes who need a kidney transplant the chance to have a pancreas transplant at the same time. In these circumstances, the results seem to be better than if a pancreas is transplanted on its own. If both transplants are successful, this is a real bonus as the recipient can stop both renal dialysis and insulin. For those who do not have kidney failure, the most promising development is an islet cell transplant (see next question).

Are there any hospitals carrying out transplants of the islets of Langerhans? Would I be able to donate my cells to my insulin-treated daughter?

Seven centres around the UK have signed up to the Diabetes UK Islet Transplantation Consortium. This group is hoping to replicate and refine the technique developed by the English surgeon, James Shapiro, and his team in Edmonton, Canada. The Edmonton team took islet cells from donor pancreases and injected them into the liver of people with Type 1 diabetes. Once in the liver the cells developed a blood supply and began producing insulin. The entire transplantation process is now known as the Edmonton Protocol.

However, it is not possible to take islets from living donors so you would be unable to donate your cells to your daughter. This technique is still in the experimental stage but the results look promising. In Edmonton, 13 out of 15 islet cell transplants were 100% successful. With time, the transplanted islets began to fail so that after one year, 33% of people needed insulin and by two years this figure was 57%. However, the transplants retain some capacity to produce insulin since most people needed to take much lower doses of insulin after the procedure. The CITR website: www.spitfire.emmes.com/study/isl/index carries this information.

Like transplantation of any other organ, an islet cell transplant requires powerful drugs to prevent rejection of the new cells (immunosuppressive therapy). As a result only people who have extreme problems in controlling their blood glucose levels are considered for transplantation. People who receive islet cell transplants need lifelong immunosuppressive drugs, which may cause long-term side effects, including various forms of cancer.

Researchers have tried to prevent the need for immunosuppressant drugs by placing the islets in a small capsule which can resist rejection while allowing insulin to pass across the membrane. Unfortunately, after a time, the membrane tends to get clogged with scar tissue and the islet graft stops working.

Until there has been a major breakthrough in the transplantation of tissues from one individual to another, the hazards of long-term immunosuppressive therapy for someone receiving either a pancreas transplant or an islet cell transplant are greater than those of having diabetes treated with insulin. The problems are not insuperable but much more research needs to be done before transplantation becomes routine treatment for Type 1 diabetes.

INSULIN PUMPS AND ARTIFICIAL PANCREAS

I recently read about a device called a 'glucose sensor', which can control the insulin administered to animals with diabetes. Will this ever be used on humans and if so what can we expect from it?

Research has been going on for many years into the development of a small electronic device that could be implanted under the skin to monitor the level of glucose in the blood continuously. The technical problems of such a device are considerable and it seems unlikely to be used routinely in people with diabetes for several years. Not only are there technical problems in achieving an accurate reflection of blood glucose level by an implanted glucose sensor, but there is also the major problem of 'hooking it up' to a supply of insulin to be released according to the blood glucose level. Clinical trials are being carried out in the USA and France using an intravenous glucose sensor in conjunction with an implantable pump. The early results are encouraging, but it will be several years before it is widely available.

I understand that there are ways of testing blood glucose without pricking the skin. Can you tell me more about them?

There are regular reports in the press about 'non-invasive' blood glucose monitoring devices being developed. Some of these devices are not totally non-invasive. One involves a needle being inserted under the skin for up to three days at a time so that blood glucose readings can be taken every few minutes. At the moment the readings given can be accessed only by a healthcare professional, but it is hoped that eventually people will be able to read these results for themselves. This method of monitoring could be useful if the device were attached to an insulin pump adjusting the amount of insulin administered in response to the blood glucose level. Although this is not yet possible, it is likely to be developed in the near future.

I hear that there are pumps available that can be implanted like pacemakers – is this true? What are the likely developments with insulin pumps within the next five years?

Yes, it is true that insulin pumps have been implanted into people as part of research studies and there has been some encouraging progress in this field. Although still experimental and a long way from being a standard form of treatment, there are pumps small enough to be implanted into the wall of the abdomen, where they remain for several years. One such pump is made by MiniMed but is very expensive and not available in the UK or USA. The pump does not have a sensor to detect glucose but simply provides background insulin at a rate that can be regulated from the outside using a small radio transmitter. This device can be used to infuse more insulin before a meal. There is a reservoir of insulin that has to be refilled through the skin with a syringe and needle but changing the batteries requires a small operation. Although it looks promising, this device is complex and expensive and remains a research procedure.

I have heard about the artificial pancreas or 'Biostator'. Apparently this machine is capable of maintaining blood glucose at normal levels, irrespective of what is eaten. Is this true? If so, why isn't it widely available?

The Biostator is an artificial pancreas, which measures the blood glucose concentration continuously and infuses insulin at a rate which keeps the blood glucose normal. Unfortunately, these machines are the size of a domestic washing machine and are technically complex. Their major value is for research purposes since they are quite unsuitable at present as devices for long-term control. The Biostator has been around for 30 years and throughout this time, bioengineering groups have tried but failed to reduce it to a size that would be practical for everyday use.

POSSIBLE DEVELOPMENTS IN INSULIN DELIVERY

What advances can we expect in the development of new insulin in the coming years?

Over the past 20 years, the range of insulins available has undergone a huge change and biosynthetic insulins have replaced the original animal insulins. There is more detail about human insulins in Chapter 3. They are manufactured by interfering with the genetic codes of bacteria and yeasts and inserting material that 'instructs' the organisms to produce insulin. By inserting the genetic material which codes for human insulin, scientists can persuade the organisms to produce human insulin. They can even get them to make 'new' analogue insulins with 'invented' structures – we are now in the era of 'designer' insulins! There is virtually unlimited capability to modify natural insulin and we expect to be able to develop a whole range of insulins with new properties that should improve therapy.

We are already beginning to see the benefits from this advance in scientific manufacturing. Analogue insulins with very rapid action are now widely used: Humalog® from Lilly and NovoRapid® from Novo Nordisk (see Table 3.1 in Chapter 3). Very long-acting analogues, Lantus® (Aventis) and Levemir® (Novo Nordisk) are now well-established.

Scientists are also looking for variations in the structure of the insulin which will 'target' the insulin more directly to the liver, the major organ responsible for glucose production in the body. Normally insulin is produced by the pancreas and goes directly to the liver but unfortunately, when people inject insulin, it has to pass through the lungs and other parts of the body before reaching the liver. It should be possible to modify the structure so that it can be targeted at the liver and control blood glucose more effectively.

I have heard that it is possible to get away from insulin injections either by using nasal insulin sprays or some form of insulin that can be taken by mouth. Are these claims true and are we going to be able to get away from insulin injections in the future?

There is no doubt that insulin delivered via the nose is absorbed through the mucous membranes and can lower the blood glucose. Unfortunately, only a small percentage of insulin taken in this manner is absorbed into the bloodstream and it is therefore an inefficient, unpredictable and expensive way of administering insulin.

If insulin is taken orally it is digested in the stomach and becomes inactive. It is possible to prevent this by incorporating insulin into a fat droplet (liposome), which enables it to be absorbed from the gut without being broken down by the digestive juices. However, the absorption is very erratic and there is no way of knowing when the insulin will be released from the droplet and become active.

Inhaled insulin (Exubera® made by Pfizer) became available in the UK in 2006 (see question under *Types of insulin* in Chapter 3). So far, the regulatory bodies have made it very difficult for people who might like to use this to obtain it, partly because it is more expensive than injected insulin. Other companies are developing different ways of giving insulin into the lungs and if they are able to price these more competitively, they are more likely to be accepted.

All these developments are exciting but there are various issues to be aware of when considering the effectiveness of inhaled and oral insulin.

- People must be confident of receiving an accurate dose of the insulin.

- Inhalers often use very large doses of insulin.

- We do not yet know the potential side effects of such large doses.

- The inhalers being developed so far do not totally eliminate the need for insulin injections because they only replace short-acting insulin: background insulin will still need to be injected.

- The devices need to be portable, compact and competitively priced.

NEW TREATMENTS

Are any new drugs becoming available for treatment of diabetes?

A new group of drugs called PKC (protein kinase C) inhibitors should be available fairly soon. These are designed to protect against long-term complications. Protein kinase C is an enzyme which becomes activated by high blood glucose levels and causes damage to the lining of small blood vessels. We know that this type of damage may lead to changes in the retina, kidney and nerves. PKC inhibitors block the action of protein kinase C and protect against these complications. Tests in people with retinopathy have shown promising results but further testing is required before they can be licensed for general use.

11 | Self-help groups

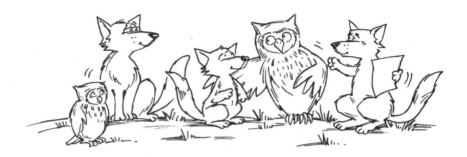

This chapter describes the various organisations that have grown up to help people with diabetes.

People react in different ways to being diagnosed with diabetes: some will become withdrawn, while others will set out to gather as much information as possible. Whatever your reaction, you should make contact with Diabetes UK, where you will come across people who are living with diabetes and who have learned to cope with many of the daily problems. These people and the staff at Diabetes UK should provide an extra dimension to the information that you have been given by doctors, nurses, dietitians and other professionals.

DIABETES UK

This organisation was founded in 1934, under the name of the British Diabetic Association, by two people with diabetes, the author HG Wells, and RD Lawrence, a doctor based at the diabetes clinic of King's College Hospital, London. In a letter to *The Times* of January 1933, they announced their intention to set up an 'association open to all diabetics, rich or poor, for mutual aid and assistance, and to promote the study, the diffusion of knowledge, and the proper treatment of diabetes in this country'. They proposed that people with diabetes, members of the general public interested in diabetes, and doctors and nurses should be persuaded to join the proposed association. Over 70 years later Diabetes UK is a credit to its founders.

In many countries there are separate organisations for people with diabetes and for professionals, but Diabetes UK draws its strength from the fact that both interest groups are united in the same society. Diabetes UK is the largest organisation in the UK working for people with diabetes, funding research, campaigning, and helping people live with the condition. The Careline offers confidential support and information on all aspects of diabetes (0845 120 2960, Monday–Friday, 9 a.m.–5 p.m.). During 2006 Careline handled an average of 200 calls each day. In order to make Careline accessible to all, there is access to an interpreting service.

Many people with diabetes experience discrimination when taking out insurance, such as increased premiums, restricted terms or even downright refusal. Faced with the general lack of understanding within the insurance market, Diabetes UK has negotiated its own exclusive schemes to provide policies suited to the needs of people with diabetes and those living with them. Diabetes UK Insurance Services offers competitively priced home, motor, travel and personal finance products. Go to the Diabetes UK website and follow 'How we help' to *Financial Services* and then *Insurance*. The current Helpline for Insurance Services is 0800 731 7431.

Up-to-date information and news is published in *Balance*, a magazine that appears every other month. 'Diabetes for beginners' is provided for newly diagnosed people, both Type 1 and Type 2 (insulin dependent and non-insulin dependent). Diabetes UK produces its own leaflets and books, and also sells books produced by other publishers; call 0800 585 088 for a catalogue (see Appendix 1). Diabetes UK has an excellent website (www.diabetes.org.uk) where you can find out more information about the work of the charity and how it can help you. Diabetes UK's address is given in Appendix 2.

Joining Diabetes UK

Diabetes UK works to influence the decisions made about living with diabetes, and the more members it has, the greater its influence. Diabetes UK cannot continue to provide its services and activities to all people with diabetes without your support. If you would like more information about joining Diabetes UK, call 0800 138 5605 or write to Diabetes UK at the address shown in Appendix 2.

Diabetes UK Local Support Groups

There are nearly 400 voluntary groups and parents' groups throughout the country. These are run entirely by volunteers and, because of their commitment, large sums of money are raised for research into diabetes. Diabetes UK branches also aim to increase public awareness of diabetes, and arrange meetings for local people with diabetes and their families for support and information.

Diabetes UK holidays

The first diabetes holidays for children in the UK took place in 1935 and running these holidays has grown into a large enterprise. During the summer of 2006, at seven different sites throughout the UK, 250 children, aged 7–18 years, enjoyed a week away with Diabetes UK. These educational holidays are organised by the Care Support team, and they give the opportunity for children to meet others with diabetes and to become more independent of their parents. They aim to give the children a good time, and encourage them to try new activities, while at the same time teaching them more about their diabetes and giving their parents a well-earned break.

Diabetes UK family weekends

The Care Support team also organises family weekends for parents of children with diabetes. These cater for about 200 families each year.

While parents have talks and discussions from specialist doctors, nurses and dietitians, there are activities for children throughout the weekend supervised by skilled and experienced helpers.

Diabetes UK adult support weekends

These weekends are for adults with diabetes who have been diagnosed in the last two or three years. They offer a chance for people with Type 1 or Type 2 diabetes to meet others, join in discussion groups, talk to healthcare professionals, and learn more about healthy eating, physical activity and care.

JUVENILE DIABETES RESEARCH FOUNDATION (JDRF)

This organisation was founded in 1970 by a small group of parents of children with diabetes. The Juvenile Diabetes Research Foundation exists to find a cure for diabetes and its complications. It supports diabetes worldwide and provides research funds at a comparable level to Diabetes UK. The address and website can be found in Appendix 2.

INSULIN-PUMPERS

This group was formed to raise funds and provide information on insulin pumps. The website address can be found in Appendix 2.

INSULIN DEPENDENT DIABETES TRUST (IDDT)

This is a registered charity formed in 1994, which is concerned with listening to the needs of people who live with diabetes. The aims of the Trust are:

- to offer care and support to people with diabetes and their

284 DIABETES: ANSWERS AT YOUR FINGERTIPS

carers, especially those experiencing difficulties with
genetically engineered 'human' insulin;

- to influence appropriate bodies to ensure that a wide range of
  insulins remains available, to ensure that all insulin users have
  a continued supply of their chosen insulin;

- to ensure that all people with diabetes and carers are properly
  informed of the various treatments available to them, as is
  their right under the Patients' Charter;

- to collect information and experiences from people with
  diabetes and their carers to help others in the same situation
  and to pass it to healthcare professionals to create a better
  understanding of 'life with diabetes';

- where possible, to represent the direct voice of the person with
  diabetes, as the consumer, in relation to healthcare and research.

The Trust is run entirely by voluntary donations and does not
accept funding from the pharmaceutical industry, in order to remain
uninfluenced and independent. The address and website can be
found in Appendix 2.

NATIONAL KIDNEY FEDERATION (NKF)

The NKF is a UK-wide charity run by kidney patients for kidney
patients. While it used to be concerned almost solely with people with
advanced or end-stage renal failure, there is emphasis now also on
people at earlier stages of kidney disease. If you have even a mild form
of kidney disease, the NKF can help you find information and support
to keep your kidneys as healthy as possible for as long as possible.

One of the long-term complications of diabetes can be some
degree of kidney damage, so it is important for people with diabetes
to be aware of this organisation and what it has to offer. The address
and website can be found in Appendix 2.

12 | Emergencies

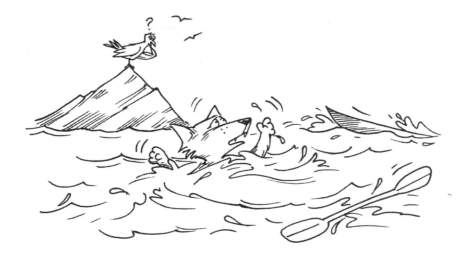

This chapter is for quick reference if things are going badly wrong. It provides vital information for people with diabetes, as well as some simple rules for relatives and friends. These rules are designed to be consulted in an emergency, although it would be worth looking through them before you are faced with a crisis. You can read more about hypos on p. 80 and about how to deal with illness on p. 147. It seems a pity to end this book in such a negative way by telling you what to do in an emergency. We hope that by keeping your diabetes well controlled you will avoid these serious situations.

WHAT EVERY PERSON ON INSULIN MUST KNOW

- *Never* stop insulin if you feel ill or sick. Illness often causes a rise in blood sugar and you may need more rather than less insulin even if you are not eating. Check your blood glucose frequently and take extra short-acting insulin every 3–4 hours if you are high. Be prepared with a high sugar drink such as Lucozade® so that if you do go low you can correct it quickly.

- If you are being sick, try to keep up a good fluid intake – at least 2½ litres (4 pints) a day. If you are unable to keep down fluids, you will need to go to hospital for an intravenous drip.

- *Always* keep sugar or some similar quick-acting carbo-hydrate on your person.

- *Never* risk driving if your blood sugar could be low. People with diabetes *do* lose their driving licence if found at the wheel when hypo.

- *Remember* physical exercise and alcohol are both likely to bring on a hypo.

WHAT OTHER PEOPLE MUST KNOW ABOUT DIABETES

- *Never* stop insulin in case of sickness (no apologies for repeating this). Check blood sugar regularly and keep a glucose drink nearby in case of hypo. Be prepared to use extra insulin if the blood tests are high.

- Repeated vomiting, drowsiness and laboured breathing are serious warning signs in someone with diabetes. They suggest impending coma and can *only* be treated in hospital.

- A person who is hypo may not be in full command of their senses and may take a lot of persuasion to have some sugar. Jam or a sugary drink (e.g. Lucozade®) may be easier to get down than Dextro-Energy tablets. Glucogel (previously known as Hypostop) which can be absorbed through the cheeks or gums may be useful.

- *Never* let someone drive if you suspect they are hypo. It could be fatal.

FOODS TO EAT IN AN EMERGENCY OR WHEN FEELING UNWELL

Each of the following contains 10 g carbohydrate.

- 100 mL pure fruit juice
- 100 mL Coca-Cola, Pepsi or similar
- 60 mL Lucozade®
- small scoop ice-cream
- two sugar cubes or two teaspoons of sugar
- one ordinary jelly cube or two heaped tablespoons of made-up jelly
- 200 mL (about ⅓ pint) of milk
- small bowl of thickened soup
- two cream crackers
- one natural yoghurt
- one diet fruit yoghurt
- one apple or pear or orange
- one small banana
- three Dextro-Energy tablets

If you are feeling unwell, eating solid foods may not be possible and you may need to rely on sweet fluids to provide the necessary carbohydrate. Liquids such as cold, defizzed (allowed to stand and go flat) cola or Lucozade® are useful if you feel sick. Do not worry about eating the exact amount of carbohydrate at the correct time but as a general rule try to eat little and often.

If you continue to vomit, *seek medical advice*.

SIGNS AND SYMPTOMS OF HYPOGLYCAEMIA AND HYPERGLYCAEMIA

Hypoglycaemia

This is **low** blood sugar, also called a hypo, a reaction or an insulin reaction. The following signs and symptoms can develop over minutes.

- Trembling
- Sweating
- Tingling of the lips and tongue
- Weakness
- Tiredness
- Sleepiness
- Hunger
- Blurred vision
- Palpitations
- Nausea
- Headache
- Mental confusion
- Unsteadiness
- Pallor
- Slurred speech
- Bad temper
- Change in behaviour
- Lack of concentration
- Unconsciousness (hypoglycaemic or insulin coma)

If possible treat the low sugar with a sweet drink followed by some food such as biscuits or a sandwich. If the person is unable to swallow, a glucagon injection or Glucogel given orally should help.

If in doubt, dial 999 and ask for paramedic help.

Hyperglycaemia

This is **high** blood sugar. The following signs and symptoms may develop over hours.

- Thirst

- Excess urine

- Nausea

- Abdominal pain

- Vomiting

- Drowsiness

- Rapid breathing

- Flushed, dry skin

- Unconsciousness (hyperglycaemic or diabetic coma)

A high blood sugar in someone who feels perfectly well is not a cause for concern. If necessary, extra short-acting insulin can be taken to bring the blood glucose down. If your blood glucose remains high after taking extra insulin, and you are feeling unwell, you may need to be treated in hospital with fluids and insulin given into a vein. If you are worried, seek medical advice.

Glossary

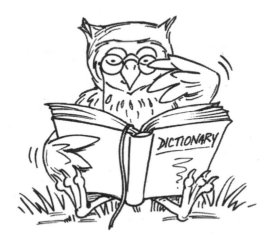

Terms in *italics* in these definitions refer to other terms in the glossary.

acetone One of the chemicals called *ketones* formed when the body uses up fat for energy. The presence of acetone in the urine usually means that more insulin is needed.

adrenaline A hormone produced by the adrenal glands, which prepares the body for action (the 'flight or fight' reaction) and also increases the level of blood glucose. Produced by the body in response to many stimuli including a low blood glucose.

albumin A protein present in most animal tissues. The presence of albumin in the urine may denote kidney damage or be simply due to a urinary infection.

alpha cell The cell that produces *glucagon* – found in the *islets of Langerhans* in the pancreas.

analogue insulin Insulin that has the molecular structure changed to alter its action.

angiography A special type of X-ray where dye is injected into an artery to detect narrowing.

angioplasty A technique which uses an inflatable balloon to widen narrowed arteries.

antigens Proteins which the body recognises as 'foreign' and which trigger an immune response.

arteriosclerosis or **arterial sclerosis** or **arterial disease** Hardening of the arteries: loss of elasticity in the walls of the arteries from thickening and calcification. Occurs with advancing years in those with or without diabetes. May affect the heart (causing thrombosis), the brain (a stroke) or the circulation to the legs and feet.

aspartame A low-calorie intense sweetener. Brand name NutraSweet®.

autonomic neuropathy Damage to the system of nerves regulating many automatic functions of the body such as stomach emptying, sexual function (potency) and blood pressure control.

bacteria A type of germ.

balanitis Inflammation of the end of the penis, usually caused by yeast infections as a result of sugar in the urine.

beta-blockers Drugs that block the effect of stress hormones on the cardiovascular system. Often used to treat angina and to lower blood pressure. May change the warning signs of *hypoglycaemia*.

beta cell The cell that produces insulin – found in the *islets of Langerhans* in the *pancreas*.

blood glucose monitoring System of measuring blood glucose levels at home using a portable meter and reagent sticks.

brittle diabetes Refers to diabetes that is very unstable with swings from very low to very high blood glucose levels and often involving frequent admissions to hospital.

calories Units in which energy or heat are measured. The energy value of food is measured in calories.

carbohydrates A class of food that comprises starches and sugars and is most readily available by the body for energy. Found mainly in plant foods. Examples are rice, bread, potatoes, pasta and beans.

cataract Opacity of the lens of the eye, which obscures vision. It may be removed surgically.

CEMACH Confidential Enquiry into Maternal and Child Health. An audit of pregnancy outcome in mothers with diabetes.

Charcot foot Swelling of the foot, sometimes leading to deformity, as a result of lack of sensation (neuropathy).

clear insulin The term used to refer to short-acting insulins. However, the two long-acting analogue insulins (Lantus® and Levemir®) are also clear so the term must be used with caution.

cloudy insulin Longer-acting insulin with fine particles of insulin bound to protamine or zinc.

coeliac disease A condition of allergy to gluten (the germ of wheat flour). Causes failure of the bowel to absorb food products normally and leads to fatty diarrhoea, weight loss and abdominal pain.

coma A form of unconsciousness from which people can be roused only with difficulty. If caused by diabetes, may be a *diabetic coma* or an *insulin coma*. See Chapter 12: Emergencies.

complications Long-term consequences of imperfectly controlled diabetes. For details see Chapter 9 .

control Usually refers to blood glucose control. The aim of good control is to achieve normal blood glucose levels (4–10 mmol/L) and HbA$_{1c}$ of 6.5–7.5%.

coronary heart disease Disease of the blood vessels supplying the heart.

cystitis Inflammation of the bladder, which usually causes frequent passing of urine, accompanied by a burning pain.

DAFNE Dose Adjustment For Normal Eating. An intensive education programme for people with Type 1 diabetes.

detemir A new insulin analogue designed to last for 24 hours and act as basal insulin. Also called Levemir®.

Dextro-Energy Glucose tablets.

diabetes insipidus A disorder of the pituitary gland accompanied by excessive urination and thirst. Nothing to do with *diabetes mellitus*.

diabetes mellitus A disorder of the pancreas characterised by a high blood glucose level. This book is about diabetes mellitus.

diabetic amyotrophy Rare condition causing pain and/or weakness of the legs from the damage to certain nerves.

diabetic coma Extreme form of *hyperglycaemia*, usually with *ketoacidosis*, causing unconsciousness.

diabetic diarrhoea A form of diabetic *autonomic neuropathy* leading to diarrhoea.

diabetic foods Food products targeted at people with diabetes, in which ordinary sugar (sucrose) is replaced with substitutes such as *fructose* or *sorbitol*. These foods are not recommended as part of your food plan.

diabetic nephropathy Kidney damage that may occur in diabetes.

diabetic neuropathy Nerve damage that may occur in diabetes.

diabetic retinopathy Eye disease that may occur in diabetes.

dietary fibre Part of plant material that resists digestion and gives bulk to the diet. Also called *fibre* or roughage.

diuretics Agents that increase the flow of urine, commonly known as water tablets.

epidural A type of anaesthetic commonly used in obstetrics. Anaesthetic solution is injected through the spinal canal to numb the lower part of the body.

erectile dysfunction Inability to achieve or maintain an erection (impotence).

fibre Another name for dietary fibre.

fructosamine Measurement of diabetes control that reflects the average blood glucose level over the previous 2–3 weeks. Similar to haemoglobin A_{1c} which averages the blood glucose over the longer period of 2–3 months.

fructose Type of sugar found naturally in fruit and honey. Since it does not require insulin for its metabolism, it is often used as a sweetener in diabetic foods.

gangrene Death of part of the body due to a very poor blood supply. Usually occurs in the feet and may require amputation.

gastroparesis Delayed emptying of the stomach as a result of autonomic neuropathy. Can lead to erratic food absorption and vomiting.

gestational diabetes Diabetes which is diagnosed during pregnancy.

glargine A new insulin analogue designed to last for 24 hours to act as basal (background) insulin. Also called Lantus®.

glaucoma Disease of the eye causing increased pressure inside the eyeball.

glucagon A hormone produced by the *alpha cells* in the pancreas which causes a rise in blood glucose by freeing *glycogen* from the liver. Available in injection form for use in treating a severe hypo.

glucose Form of sugar made by digestion of carbohydrates. Absorbed into the bloodstream where it circulates and is used as a source of energy.

glucose tolerance test Test used in the diagnosis of diabetes mellitus. The glucose in the blood is measured at intervals before and after the person has drunk a large amount of glucose while fasting.

gluten sensitivity The underlying cause of *coeliac disease.* This is more common in people with Type 1 diabetes.

glycogen The form in which carbohydrate is stored in the liver and muscles. It is often known as animal starch.

glycaemic index (GI) A way of describing how a carbohydrate-containing food affects blood glucose levels.

glycosuria Presence of glucose in the urine.

glycosylated haemoglobin Another name for haemoglobin A_{1c}.

haemoglobin A_{1c} The part of the haemoglobin or pigment of the red blood cell which has glucose attached to it. A test of diabetes control. The amount of haemoglobin A_{1c} in the blood depends on the average blood glucose level over the previous 2–3 months.

honeymoon period Time when the dose of insulin drops shortly after starting insulin treatment. It is the result of partial recovery of insulin secretion by the pancreas. Usually the honeymoon period only lasts for a few months.

hormone Substance generated in one gland or organ which is carried by the blood to another part of the body to control another organ. Insulin and glucagon are both hormones.

human insulin Insulin that has been manufactured to be identical to that produced in the human pancreas. Differs slightly from older insulins, which were extracted from cows or pigs.

hydramnios An excessive amount of amniotic fluid, which is the fluid surrounding the baby before birth.

hyperglycaemia High blood glucose (above 10 mmol/L).

hypo Abbreviation for hypoglycaemia.

hypoglycaemia (also known as a hypo or an insulin reaction) Low blood glucose (below 3.5 mmol/L).

impotence Failure of erection of the penis.

injector Device to aid injections.

Innolet A simple injector for insulin designed for people with poor vision or problems with their hands such as arthritis.

insulin A hormone produced by the *beta cells* of the pancreas and responsible for control of blood glucose. Insulin can only be given by injection because digestive juices destroy its action if taken by mouth.

insulin coma Extreme form of *hypoglycaemia* associated with unconsciousness and sometimes convulsions.

insulin dependent diabetes (abbreviation IDD) Former name for Type 1 diabetes.

insulin pen Device that resembles a large fountain pen that takes a cartridge of insulin. The injection of insulin is given after dialling the dose and pressing a button that releases the insulin.

insulin reaction Another name for *hypoglycaemia* or a hypo. In America it is called an insulin shock.

insulin resistance A condition where the normal amount of insulin is not able to keep the blood glucose level down to normal. Such people need large doses of insulin to control their diabetes.

intermediate-acting insulin Insulin preparations with action lasting 12–18 hours.

intradermal Meaning 'into the skin'. Usually refers to an injection given into the most superficial layer of the skin. Insulin must not be given in this way as it is painful and will not be absorbed properly (see Figure 3.3).

intramuscular A deep injection into the muscle.

islets of Langerhans Specialised cells within the pancreas that produce *insulin* and *glucagon*.

isophane A form of intermediate-acting insulin that has protamine added to slow its absorption.

joule Unit of work or energy used in the metric system. A *calorie* is equivalent to about 4.18 joules. Some dietitians calculate food energy in joules.

juvenile-onset diabetes Outdated name for Type 1 diabetes, so-called because most people receiving insulin develop diabetes under the age of 40. The term is no longer used because Type 1 diabetes can occur at any age, although more commonly in young people.

ketoacidosis A serious condition caused by lack of insulin which results in body fat being used up to form *ketones* and acids. Characterised by high blood glucose levels, ketones in the urine, vomiting, drowsiness, heavy laboured breathing and a smell of acetone on the breath.

ketones Acid substances (including acetone) formed when body fat is used up to provide energy.

ketonuria The presence of *acetone* and other ketones in the urine. Detected by testing with a special testing stick (Ketostix®, Ketur Test®). Presence of ketones in the urine is due to lack of insulin or periods of starvation.

laser treatment Process in which laser beams are used to treat a damaged retina (back of the eye). Used in *photocoagulation*.

lente insulin A form of intermediate-acting insulin that has zinc added to slow its absorption. It is now obsolete and very few people use this insulin.

lipoatrophy Loss of fat from injection sites. It used to occur before the use of highly purified insulins.

lipohypertrophy Fatty swelling usually caused by repeated injections of insulin into the same site.

maturity-onset diabetes Another term for Type 2 diabetes most commonly occurring in people who are middle-aged and overweight.

metabolic rate Rate of oxygen consumption by the body; rate at which you 'burn up' the food you eat.

metabolism Process by which the body turns food into energy.

microalbuminuria Small amounts of protein in the urine, not detectable by dipstick for albumin (*proteinuria*). Raised levels indicate early kidney damage.

microaneurysms Small red dots on the retina at the back of the eye which are one of the earliest signs of diabetic *retinopathy*. They represent areas of weakness of the very small blood vessels in the eye. Microaneurysms do not affect the eyesight in any way.

micromole One-thousandth (1/1000) of a millimole.

millimole Unit for measuring the concentration of glucose and other substances in the blood. Blood glucose is measured in millimoles per litre (mmol/L). It has replaced milligrammes per decilitre (mg/dL or mg%) as a unit of measurement although this is still used in some other countries. 1 mmol/L = 18 mg/dL.

nephropathy Kidney damage. In the first instance this makes the kidney more leaky so that *albumin* appears in the urine. At a later stage it may affect the function of the kidney and in severe cases lead to kidney failure.

neuropathy Damage to the nerves, which may be *peripheral* neuropathy or *autonomic neuropathy*. It can occur with diabetes especially when poorly controlled, but also has other causes.

NICE National Institute for Health and Clinical Excellence. An independent organisation providing national guidance to promote good health. It provides guidelines for the use of new and existing drugs in the NHS.

non-insulin dependent diabetes (abbreviation NIDD) Former name for Type 2 diabetes.

orlistat A tablet that blocks the digestion of fat. Brand name Xenical®. Used to help people lose weight, which in turn may improve control of diabetes.

pancreas Gland lying behind the stomach, which as well as secreting a digestive fluid (pancreatic juice) also produces the hormones *insulin* and *glucagon*. Contains *islets of Langerhans*.

peripheral neuropathy Damage to the nerves supplying the muscles and skin. This can result in diminished sensation, particularly in the feet and legs, and in muscle weakness. May also cause pain in the feet or legs.

pernicious anaemia An autoimmune condition which causes failure of the body to absorb vitamin B12, which is a vital constituent of haemoglobin – the main component of red blood cells. In the absence of B12, red blood cells fail to develop normally and the patient becomes anaemic. Like many autoimmune conditions, it is more common in Type 1 diabetes.

phimosis Inflammation and narrowing of the foreskin of the penis.

photocoagulation Process of treating diabetic retinopathy with light beams, either laser beams or xenon arc. This technique focuses a beam of light on a very tiny area of the retina. This beam is so intense that it causes a very small burn, which may close off a leaking blood vessel or destroy weak blood vessels that are at risk of bleeding.

PKC inhibitors (protein kinase C inhibitors) Developed to try and reverse the changes in small blood vessels which cause diabetic eye disease (retinopathy). Though they seem to help in isolated cases, overall the results have been disappointing.

polydipsia Being excessively thirsty and drinking too much. It is a symptom of untreated diabetes.

polyuria The passing of large quantities of urine due to excess glucose from the bloodstream. It is a symptom of untreated diabetes.

pork insulin Insulin extracted from the pancreas of pigs.

pre-eclampsia A condition which occurs towards the end of pregnancy and leads to high blood pressure, protein in the urine and in severe cases, convulsions. Pre-eclampsia normally resolves soon after delivery.

protein One of the classes of food that is necessary for growth and repair of tissues. Found in fish, meat, eggs, milk and pulses. Can also refer to albumin when found in the urine.

proteinuria Protein or albumin in the urine.

pruritus vulvae Irritation of the vulva (the genital area in women). Caused by an infection that occurs because of an excess of sugar in the urine and is often an early sign of diabetes in the older person. It clears up when the blood glucose levels return to normal and the sugar disappears from the urine.

pyelonephritis Inflammation and infection of the kidney.

renal threshold The level of glucose in the blood above which it will begin to spill into the urine. The usual renal threshold for glucose in the blood is about 10 mmol/L, so when the blood glucose rises above 10 mmol/L, glucose appears in the urine.

retina Light-sensitive area at the back of the eye.

retinal screening Photograph of the retina to identify changes due to diabetes at a stage that they can be treated to prevent loss of vision. Usually carried out once a year.

retinopathy Damage to the retina.

rimonabant New drug designed to help obese people by reducing appetite. May also help people give up smoking, though it is not licensed for this. It is not yet available in the NHS and is being evaluated by NICE. Also named Acomplia®.

roughage Another name for dietary fibre.

saccharin A synthetic sweetener that is calorie free.

short-acting insulin Insulin preparations with action lasting 6–8 hours.

Snellen chart Chart showing rows of letters in decreasing sizes. Used for measuring visual acuity.

sorbitol A chemical related to sugar and alcohol that is used as a sweetening agent in foods as a substitute for ordinary sugar. It has no significant effect upon the blood glucose level but has the same number of calories as ordinary sugar so should not be used by those who need to lose weight. Poorly absorbed and may have a laxative effect.

steroids Hormones produced by the adrenal glands, testes and ovaries. Also available in synthetic form. Tend to increase the blood glucose level and make diabetes worse.

subcutaneous injection An injection beneath the skin into the layer of fat that lies between the skin and muscle. The normal way of giving insulin.

sucrose A sugar (containing glucose and fructose in combination) derived from sugar cane or sugar beet (i.e. ordinary table sugar). It is a pure carbohydrate.

thrombosis Clot forming in a blood vessel.

thyroid gland Situated in the neck, this gland controls the rate of metabolism. An overactive thyroid (thyrotoxicosis) causes a rapid heart rate, disturbed sleep, increased appetite and anxiety but also tiredness. An underactive thyroid leads to sluggishness and weight increase. Both conditions are more common in Type 1 diabetes.

tissue markers Proteins on the outside of cells in the body that are genetically determined.

MORECAMBE BAY HOSPITALS NHS TRUST

toxaemia Poisoning of the blood by the absorption of toxins. Usually refers to the toxaemia of pregnancy, which is characterised by high blood pressure, proteinuria and ankle swelling.

Type 1 diabetes Name for insulin dependent diabetes which cannot be treated by diet and tablets alone. Outdated name is juvenile-onset diabetes. Age of onset is usually below the age of 40 years.

Type 2 diabetes Name for non-insulin dependent diabetes. Age of onset is usually above the age of 40 years, often in people who are overweight. These people do not always need insulin treatment and can usually be successfully treated with diet alone or diet and tablets. Formerly known as maturity-onset diabetes.

U40 insulin The old weaker strength of insulin, no longer available in the UK. It is still available in Eastern Europe and in some countries in the Far East, such as Vietnam and Indonesia.

U100 insulin The standard strength of insulin in the UK, USA, Canada, Australia, New Zealand, South Africa, the Middle East and the Far East.

urine testing The detection of abnormal amounts of glucose, ketones, protein or blood in the urine, usually by means of urine-testing sticks.

virus A very small organism capable of causing disease.

viscous fibre A type of dietary fibre found in pulses (peas, beans and lentils) and some fruit and vegetables.

visual acuity Acuteness of vision. Measured by reading letters on a sight-testing chart (a Snellen chart).

vitiligo A skin condition, more common in people with Type 1 diabetes and thyroid disease, in which areas of skin (mainly the back of hands, face and neck) lose pigment (melanin) and the surrounding skin often becomes over-pigmented. The patches of depigmentation enlarge slowly with time. There is no specific treatment but areas of vitiligo must be protected from sun damage with high factor UV products.

water tablets The common name for diuretics.

Xenical The brand name for orlistat.

Appendix 1: Publications

At the time of writing, all the publications listed here were available. Check with your local bookshop or Diabetes UK for current prices.

ABOUT DIABETES

Books

Type 1 Diabetes in Children, Adolescents and Young Adults by Ragnar Hanas. Class (2006)

Need to Know: Diabetes (Need to Know) by Jenny Bryan. Heinemann (2004)

Diabetes and Your Teenager by Bonnie Estridge and Jo Davies. Harper Collins (1996)

Magazines and booklets

These titles are all published by Diabetes UK.

Balance – Diabetes UK's own magazine which appears every other month

Diabetes for Beginners: Type 1

Diabetes for Beginners: Type 2

What Diabetes Care to Expect

Living Healthily with Diabetes – a guide for Black African-Caribbean communities

Coping with diabetes when you are ill

NUTRITION

Apart from the books listed here, you will also be able to find other titles in your local library or on Amazon.

Books

The Everyday Diabetic Cookbook by Stella Bowling. Grub Street Publishing (1995)

The Good Housekeeping Diabetic Cookbook by Azmina Govindji. Collins & Brown (2005)

Leaflets

These are available from Diabetes UK, some as downloads.

Food choices and diabetes

Eating well with diabetes

Alcohol and diabetes

Recipe books

These titles are all published by Diabetes UK.

The Diabetes Weight Loss Diet

Home Baking

Managing your weight – a balanced approach

Christmas and other celebrations

Quick cooking for diabetes

Appendix 2: Useful addresses

AccuChek
Customer careline:
Freephone Tel: 0800 701 000
*Insulin pumps and blood glucose
meters*

A Menarini Diagnostics
Tel: 01189 444 100
Website: www.menarinidiag.co.uk
Blood glucose meters

Aventis Pharma
Tel: 01732 584000
Website: www.aventis.com

Bayer
Helpline: 01635 566366
Website: www.bayer.co.uk
*Pharmaceutical company
Manufactures blood glucose meters
and provides helpline*

Becton, Dickinson & Co
Tel: 01865 748844
Website: www.bddiabetes.com
*Manufactures insulin pens, syringes
and needles and provides helpline*

Bio-Diagnostics
Tel: 01684 592262
Website: www.bio-diagnostics.co.uk
Supplier of Glucogel

British Heart Foundation (BHF)
Helpline: 08450 708070
Website: www.bhf.org.uk
*Funds research, promotes education
and raises money to buy equipment
to treat people with heart disease.
For list of publications, posters and
videos, send s.a.e. Their helpline,
HeartstartUK, can arrange training
in emergency life-saving techniques for
lay people*

British Hypertension Society
Tel: 020 8979 8300
Website: www.hamptonmedical.com

British Parachute Association
Tel: 01162 785271
Website: www.bpa.org.uk
*Governing body of sport parachuting.
Offers medical assessment on
suitability for parachuting to people
with medical disorders*

British Sub-Aqua Club
Tel: 01513 506200
Website: www.bsac.com
*Governing body for sub-aqua sport.
Offers medical assessment for those
with medical disorders wanting to take
part in diving underwater*

CDx Ltd
Helpline: 0191 564 2036
Website: www.cdx.uk.com
Maker of SensoCard Plus, a talking blood glucose meter

CP Pharmaceuticals
Now merged to form Wockhardt UK

Cygnus UK
Previously supplied Glucowatch, a continuous blood glucose monitor. There were a number of technical problems and Glucowatch has now been withdrawn

Department of Health (DoH)
Helpline: 0800 555777
Produces and distributes literature about public health. National Service Framework for Diabetes can be obtained from:
www. doh.gov.uk/nsf/diabetes.htm

Diabetes Research and Wellness Foundation
Tel: 02392 637 08
Website: www.diabeteswellnessnet.org.uk
A diabetes support organisation based in Washington DC, USA with a base in the UK. Funds medical research; its membership receive newsletters with personal stories and question and answer section

Diabetes UK
10 Parkway
London NW1 7AA
Helpline: 020 7424 1030/1000
Fax: 020 7424 1001
Textline: 020 7424 1888
Website: www.diabetes.org.uk
Provides advice and information on diabetes; has local support groups

DiagnoSys Medical
Helpline: 0800 08 588 08
Distributors of blood glucose monitors and a range of other products via mail order

Diesetronic Medical Systems
This pump manufacturer has been taken over by the American giant Roche, which now supplies insulin pumps under the name AccuChek

Disability Alliance
Helpline: 020 7247 8763
Website: www.disabilityalliance.org
Produces the Disability Rights Handbook. *Updated three times a year, it addresses every aspect of social services benefits for people with disabilities. Offers advice on benefits and training for other organisations and is involved with policy issues*

**The Guide Dogs
for the Blind Association**
Tel: 0870 600 2323
Website: www.guidedogs@gdba.org.uk
*Provides guide dogs, mobility and
other rehabilitation services that
enable blind and partially sighted
people to lead the fullest and most
independent lives possible*

Health Development Agency
*Formerly Health Education Authority
and now taken over by NICE*

Heart UK
7 North Road
Maidenhead SL6 1PE
Tel: 01628 628638
Fax: 01628 628698
Website: www.heartuk.org.uk
*Will help anyone at high risk of heart
attack, but specialises in inherited
conditions causing high cholesterol
(familial hypercholesterolaemia)*

HeartstartUK
see under British Heart Foundation

The Impotence Association
see under The Sexual Dysfunction
Association

Insulin Dependent Diabetes Trust
Tel: 01604 622837
Website: www.iddtinternational.org
*Trust set up to help and advise people
having problems with human insulin.
Collects insulin for distribution in
developing countries. Also runs
Sponsor a child scheme for a clinic
in India*

Insulin-Pumpers UK
Website: www.insulin-pumpers.org.uk.
*Offers information on the use of
pumps and puts people in touch with
each other. Advises on obtaining
funding if pumps are not available
via the NHS*

John Bell & Croyden
50–54 Wigmore Street
London W1U 2AU
Tel: 020 7935 5555
Website: www.johnbellcroyden.co.uk
*Dispensing pharmacy that can obtain
medicines not manufactured in the
UK, with appropriate named patient
prescription and import licence*

**Juvenile Diabetes
Research Foundation**
Tel: 020 7713 2030
Website: www.jdrf.org.uk
*Dedicated to funding research to find
a cure for Type 1 diabetes. Provides
information on the progress of
research via leaflets, newsletters
and open meetings*

LifeScan
Helpline: 0800 121200
Website: www.lifescan.com
*Manufactures blood glucose
monitoring systems and meters and
offers advice*

Eli Lilly Diabetes Care Division
Helpline: 0800 850777
Website: www.lilly.com
*Pharmaceutical company. Offers
helpline to people with diabetes*

MedicAlarm
The Old Barn
Court Farm
Overstone
Northamptonshire NN6 0AP
Tel: 01604 646200
Email: sales@medicalarm.co.uk

Medic-Alert Foundation
Helpline: 0800 581420
Website: www.medicalert.org.uk
*Offers a body-worn identification
system for people with hidden medical
conditions. Offers selection of
jewellery with internationally
recognised medical symbol. Has
24-hour emergency telephone number*

MediSense Britain
Helpline: 0500 467466
Order line: 0845 607 3247
Website: www.abbottlaboratories.com
*Manufactures blood glucose
monitoring systems and meters, and
provides information*

Medtronic
Tel: 01923 212213
Website: www.medtronic.co.uk

**NICE
The National Institute
for Health and Clinical Excellence**
11 Strand
London WC2N 5HR
Website: www. nice.org.uk

National Kidney Federation
Helpline: 0845 601 0209
Website: www.kidney.org.uk
*Provides information, campaigns for
improvement in care and supports
people through its network of local
groups*

Novo Nordisk Pharmaceuticals
Helpline: 0845 600 5055
Website: www.novonordisk.co.uk
*Manufactures injecting pens for
diabetes, growth hormone and HRT
injections*

Nutech International Ltd
Tel: 01798 865882
Website: www.nutech-international.com
*Supplier of the Lasette, a laser device
for obtaining blood for testing*

Owen Mumford
Helpline: 0800 731 6959
Website: www.owenmumford.com
*Manufactures medical products for
diabetics*

Roche Diagnostics
Helpline: 0800 701000
Website: www.roche.com
Manufactures blood glucose
monitoring systems and insulin
pumps under the name AccuChek.
Offers advice

The Royal National Institute
of the Blind
105 Judd Street
London WC1H 9NE
Helpline: 0845 766 9999
Tel: 020 7388 1266
Fax: 020 7388 2034
Website: www.rnib.org.uk
Offers a range of information and
advice on lifestyle changes and
employment for people facing loss of
sight. Also offers support and training
in braille. Mail order catalogue of
useful aids

Sanofi-Aventis
1 Onslow Street
Guildford
Surrey GU1 4YS
Tel: 01483 505515
Website: www.sanofi-aventis.co.uk

Servier Laboratories
Tel: 01753 662744
Manufactures diabetes meters, offers
advice

Sexual Dysfunction Association
2–4 Windmill Lane
Southall
Middlesex UB2 4NJ
Tel: 0807743571
Website: www.sda.uk.net
Offers a listening ear and information
on currently prescribed treatment and
how sufferers should proceed to get
best advice. Can advise on local
specialists in erectile dysfunction

SOS Talisman
106–108 Vyse Street
Hockley
Birmingham
B18 6LP
Tel: 0121 233 7455
Website: www.allertag.com

Stroke Association
Helpline: 0845 303 3100
Website: www.stroke.org.uk
Funds research and provides
information, specialising in stroke only

Sydney University's Glycaemic Index Research Service (SUGiRS)
Human Nutrition Unit
Department of Biochemistry
GO8 Sydney University
New South Wales, 2006, Australia
Tel: 0061 2 9351 3757
Fax: 0061 2 9351 6022
Website: www.glycemicindex.com
Commercial research and advisory service that measures GI values for foods, drinks and nutritional supplements. Provides advice to manufacturers to assist them in making low-GI products

Therasense
Customer Service line:
0800 138 5467
www.therasense.com
Manufactures blood glucose meters

Wockhardt UK
Tel: 01978 661261
Website: www.wockhardt.co.uk
Committed to the production of porcine and bovine insulin

Index

Numbers in *italic* indicate pages
with an illustration; those followed
by italic *g* refer to glossary entries.

eyes, laser treatment
(photocoagulation) *see under*
laser treatment, eyes
eyesight, poor 242

fasting and diabetes 133–4
feet:
    care during winter 249–50
    Charcot foot 251
    Feet Facts/Foot Care Rules
        246–7, 251, *252–3*
    foot screening 140
    foot spas 171
    foot ulcers 167, 250, 251
    going barefoot 249
    identifying potential impact of
        diabetes on 248
    inspecting 243, 245–6, 247
    problems with 243ff
    swelling of 251
    toenail cutting 244, 246
female orgasm and diabetes 172
fertility and diabetes 185
first aid 253
fludrocortisone 266
flying and diabetes *142*
folic acid 190, 195, 196
food:
    and emergencies *288*
    children and 204–5, *206–7*
    food plan 28
    guidelines *22*
    nutritional value *21*
Foot Care Rules/Feet Facts *246–7*,
    251, *252–3*
FreeStyle Freedom and Freestyle
    Mini 110
fructosamine 115, 294*g*

fructose 19, 294*g*
fruit juice, natural sugars in 29
fungicide 171

gabapentin 257
gangrene 154, 229, 243, 248,
    264, 294*g*
    possibilities of 243–4, 248
gastroparesis 260, 294*g*
genetic component to diabetes
    270–3
gestational diabetes 294*g*
ginseng and diabetes 36
glargine (Lantus) 45, 53, 54, 55,
    294*g*
glasses and diabetes 234–5
glaucoma 241, 295*g*
glibenclamide 202
GLP-1 295*g*
glucagon 2, 86, 134, 136, 290,
    291*g*, 294*g*, 296*g*
Glucogel (previously Hypostop) 87,
    134, 218, 287, 290
glucose 13, 86, 87, 134, 294*g*,
    301*g*
    high 90, 215
glucose sensor 275
glucose tolerance test 113–14, 295*g*
GlucoWatch 108
gluten sensitivity 294*g*
glycaemic control, poor 48
glycaemic index (GI) 71–72, 295*g*
glycogen 294*g*
glycosuria 295*g*
glycosylated haemoglobin (HbA$_{1c}$),
    haemoglobin A$_{1c}$ 49, 89, 91,
    96–7, 98, 107–8, 113, 114ff,
    125–6, 140, 262, 295*g*

Novo Nordisk 44, 45, 46, 47, 62, 63, 65, 69–70, 277, 306
Novopen 65
NovoRapid *see* aspart
NSF *see* National Service Framework
Nutech International 111, 306
nystatin 171

obesity
  central, definition of 27
  and children 224, 225, *226*
oedema 254
OneTouch Ultra 110
optician 14, 235, 238, 242
OptiClik Pen 62
Optium meter 112
oral contraceptives 102, 173
oral hypoglycaemic agents (OHAs) 48
Orbach, Susie 205
orlistat (Xenical) 32, 79–80, 297*g*
orthotis 250
osteoporosis 183, 184, 251
Owen Mumford (Medical Shop) *63*, 66, 103, 105
  Autopens 64, 65

pancreas 2, 39, 59, 278, 291*g*, 293*g*, 295*g*, 296*g*, 297*g*, 299*g*, 300*g*
  and antibody component to diabetes 271
  artificial 109, 275, 276–7
  babies' during gestation 182, 197
  hormones produced by 2–3, 86
  insulin production 4, 39, 56, 58, 64, 73, 271, 276

insulin failure 6
location of *2*
pregnancy and 8
transplant 273, 274, 275
see also 'Biostator', insulin, islets of Langerhans
pancreatitis 8
papaverine 178
Patients' Charter 284
PCT *see* Primary Care Trust
PenMate 62, 65
peripheral neuropathy 298*g*
pernicious anaemia 9, 298*g*
Pfizer 278
phimosis 14, 298*g*
photocoagulation *see* laser treatment
PKC inhibitors (protein kinase C inhibitors) 279, 298*g*
podiatrist 243, 244, 245, 250, 264, 265
polydipsia 298*g*
polyuria 298*g*
poor circulation and diabetes 261
pork insulin *see under* insulin
pre-eclampsia 298*g*
pregabalin 257
pregnancy and diabetes 8, 179, 180–1 184, Chapter 7, 262–3, 299*g*, 300*g*
  antenatal care 187–8
  and cholesterol/blood pressure tablets 262–3
  diabetes and complications 186, 195
  effects of poor control 186–7
  fertility 185
  and ketones 112
  and large babies 190–2

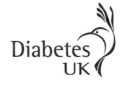

Diabetes UK

Become a member of Diabetes UK today

• •

Join Diabetes UK today to benefit from our bi-monthly members magazine, *Balance*, a network of support groups across the UK and confidential information and support from our Careline

To join today visit www.diabetes.org.uk/join

Or call 0800 138 5605

Please get in touch with us

Diabetes UK Careline is here to help. Call **0845 120 2960** for support and information. (Calls cost no more than 4p per minute, calls from mobiles usually cost more)

• •

The charity for people with diabetes
www.diabetes.org.uk
Registered charity no. 215199   009A01026

Have you found *Type 1 Diabetes: Answers at your fingertips* useful and practical? If so, you may be interested in other books from Class Publishing.

TYPE 1 DIABETES IN CHILDREN, ADOLESCENTS AND YOUNG ADULTS
£19.99

Dr Ragnar Hanas

If you have diabetes, you need to become better informed than the average doctor. Dr Hanas shows you, step-by-step, how to become an expert in your own diabetes. This remarkable book gives you all the strategies, tips and tricks to get your blood glucose down and keep it under control. It tells you everything you need to know to take good care of your condition, and live a full, healthy and happy life – controlling your diabetes rather than being controlled by it.

'This extraordinary book . . . will help you to understand diabetes better'
DR PETER SWIFT, Consultant Paediatrician, Leicester Royal Infirmary.

BEATING DEPRESSION
£17.99

Dr Stefan Cembrowicz and Dr Dorcas Kingham

Depression is one of the most common illnesses in the world – affecting up to one in four people at some time in their lives. This book shows sufferers and their families that they are not alone, and offers tried and tested techniques for overcoming depression.

'All you need to know about depression, presented in a clear, concise and readable way.'
ANN DAWSON, World Health Organization

ACNE
Answers at your fingertips
£17.99

Dr Tim Mitchell and Alison Dudley

Acne is the most common chronic skin condition of adolescents, affecting almost all to some extent. It tends to begin at puberty, and while for most people it tends to go away by the time they reach their mid-20s, a few continue to have acne for longer.

'By far the best book I have read on the subject.'
PETER LAPSLEY, Chief Executive, Skin Care Campaign

ASTHMA
Answers at your fingertips
£17.99

Dr Mark Levy, Trisha Weller and Professor Sean Hilton

Asthma – the 'at your fingertips' guide contains over 250 real questions from people with asthma and their families – answered by three medical experts. This handbook contains up-to-date, medically accurate and practical advice on living with asthma.

'A helpful and clearly written book.'
DR MARTYN PARTRIDGE, Chief Medical Adviser, National Asthma Campaign

HEART HEALTH
Answers at your fingertips
£14.99

Dr Graham Jackson

This practical handbook, written by a leading cardiologist, answers all your questions about heart conditions. It tells you all about you and your heart; how to keep your heart healthy, or if it has been affected by heart disease – how to make it as strong as possible.

'Those readers who want to know more about the various treatments for heart disease will be much enlightened.'
DR JAMES LE FANU, The Daily Telegraph

ECZEMA
Answers at your fingertips
£14.99

Dr Tim Mitchell and Alison Hepplewhite

With answers to hundreds of questions on every aspect of living with eczema, this book will help you find ways to manage your own eczema – or that of your child – to fit in with everyday interests and activities.

'What a joy to have a new book which is medically accurate, wide ranging and practical in its approach.'
MARGARET COX, Chief Executive, National Eczema Society

PRIORITY ORDER FORM

Cut out or photocopy this form and send it (post free in the UK) to:

Class Publishing   **Tel: 01256 302 699**
FREEPOST 16705   **Fax: 01256 812 558**
Macmillan Distribution
Basingstoke RG21 6ZZ

Please send me urgently   *Post included*
(tick below)   *price per copy (UK only)*

☐ **Type 1 Diabetes: Answers at your fingertips** (ISBN 978 1 85959 175 8)   £20.99

☐ **Type 1 Diabetes in Children, Adolescents and Young Adults**   £23.99
   (ISBN 978 1 85959 153 6)

☐ **Beating Depression** (ISBN 978 1 85959 150 5)   £20.99

☐ **Acne: Answers at your fingertips** (ISBN 978 1 85959 073 7)   £20.99

☐ **Asthma: Answers at your fingertips** (ISBN 978 1 85959 111 6)   £20.99

☐ **Heart Health: Answers at your fingertips** (ISBN 978 1 85959 097 3)   £17.99

☐ **Eczema: Answers at your fingertips** (ISBN 978 1 85959 125 3)   £17.99

TOTAL _____

Easy ways to pay

Cheque: I enclose a cheque payable to Class Publishing for £ _____

Credit card: Please debit my   ☐ Mastercard   ☐ Visa   ☐ Amex

Number _____ Expiry date _____

Name _____

My address for delivery is _____

_____

Town _____ County _____ Postcode _____

Telephone number (*in case of query*) _____

Credit card billing address if different from above _____

_____

Town _____ County _____ Postcode _____

Class Publishing's guarantee: remember that if, for any reason, you are not satisfied with these books, we will refund all your money, without any questions asked. Prices and VAT rates may be altered for reasons beyond our control.